"This is an impressive book of high relevance for the general audience. Social traumata – from marital and family violence, from rapes to warfare – burrow deeply into psychic structure, personal and group identity, into our ability to learn and love and to enjoy new experiences. Violence makes people silent. Primo Levi's horrific experience was that no ear wanted to listen what had been done to him in Auschwitz. Being silenced is a new social trauma. This book valuably contributes to the task to open public reception and therapeutic ears to what has been silenced – it's a must-read for the future of the helping professions."

Michael B. Buchholz, Professor, International Psychoanalytic University, Berlin, Germany

"First delivered in 2018, these selected psychoanalytic reflections on the problem of social trauma are needed even more urgently in 2022. Focused on the clinical aspects of working with persons who have experienced the acute pain of forced immigration, separation, and loss (and many more), in both individual and group forms of treatment, this book will be necessary to everyone engaged in psychoanalytic psychotherapy – as a guideline, as inspiration, and as a source of support."

Aleksandar Dimitrijevic, PhD, International Psychoanalytic University, Berlin, Germany

A Psychoanalytic Exploration of Social Trauma

A Psychoanalytic Exploration of Social Trauma presents a thorough introduction to social trauma from a range of perspectives, exploring several key themes, specific causes and symptoms and clinical interventions.

With chapters from a diverse range of authors, the book considers social trauma as it relates to stories and history, group identity, the consulting room, migration, and post-traumatic conditions. These topics are explored via a range of frames, including individual therapy, group analysis, social dream matrix, large groups, case studies, narrative recollections, and cinematographic expression. The book also considers the implications of new technology in causing and treating social trauma.

A Psychoanalytic Exploration of Social Trauma will be of great interest to psychoanalytic psychotherapists in practice and in training, psychoanalysts, and psychoanalytically informed professionals working with trauma.

Cristina Călărășanu is a psychoanalytic psychotherapist based in Romania. She is president of the Romanian Association for the Psychoanalysis of Group and Family Links, IACFP (International Association of Couple and Family Psychoanalysis) General Secretary and Scientific Council Member, EFPP (European Federation of Psychoanalytic Psychotherapy) Board Member and Chair of the Couple and Family Section.

Ulrich Schultz-Venrath is Professor of Psychosomatic Medicine and Psychotherapy at the University of Witten/Herdecke, Germany, and a psychoanalyst and training group analyst, working in private practice in Cologne, Germany. Until March 2021, he was chair of the group section of EFPP.

Hansjorg Messner is a psychoanalytic psychotherapist in private practice in London, UK. He is a senior member of the BPF (British Psychoanalytic Council) and BPC (British Psychotherapy Foundation), as well as Vice President and Chair of the adult section in the EFPP and board member of the federation.

The EFPP Monograph series

Series Editor: Cristina Călărăşanu

A series of Monographs produced in conjunction with the European Federation for Psychoanalytic Psychotherapy (EFPP). Each volume brings together writings on a particular topic by authors from several European countries. The EFPP promotes communication and discussion between psychotherapists across national boundaries in the child and adolescent, adult, family and group sections of the organisation through its conferences and seminars on topics of interest in contemporary psychoanalytic psychotherapy. The organisation represents some 13,000 psychoanalytic psychotherapists in twenty-two countries in Western, Central and Eastern Europe and is concerned with many matters which are relevant to the profession, such as training and registration.

Recent titles in the series include:

Psychoanalytic Psychotherapy of the Severely Disturbed Adolescent
Edited by Dimitris Anastasopoulos, Margot Waddell and Effie Lignos

Families in Transformation
A Psychoanalytic Approach
Edited by Anna Maria Nicolò, Pierre Benghozi and Daniela Lucarelli

A Psychoanalytic Exploration of Social Trauma
The Inner Worlds of Outer Realities
Edited by Cristina Călărăşanu, Ulrich Schultz-Venrath and Hansjorg Messner

For further information about this series please visit: https://www.routledge.com/The-EFPP-Monograph-Series/book-series/KARNACEFPPPM

A Psychoanalytic Exploration of Social Trauma

The Inner Worlds of Outer Realities

Cristina Călărășanu,
Ulrich Schultz-Venrath and
Hansjorg Messner

Routledge
Taylor & Francis Group
LONDON AND NEW YORK

Designed cover image: Getty Images | FORGEM.

First published 2023
by Routledge
4 Park Square, Milton Park, Abingdon, Oxon OX14 4RN

and by Routledge
605 Third Avenue, New York, NY 10158

Routledge is an imprint of the Taylor & Francis Group, an informa business

British Library Cataloguing-in-Publication Data
A catalogue record for this book is available from the British Library

Library of Congress Cataloging-in-Publication Data
Names: Călărăşanu, Cristina, editor. | Schultz-Venrath, Ulrich, 1952-editor. | Messner, Hansjorg, editor.
Title: A psychoanalytic exploration of social trauma : the inner worlds of outer realities / edited by Cristina Călărăşanu, Ulrich Schultz-Venrath and Hansjorg Messner.
Description: Milton Park, Abingdon, Oxon ; New York, NY : Routledge, 2023. | Series: The EFPP monograph series | Includes bibliographical references and index. |
Identifiers: LCCN 2022031620 (print) | LCCN 2022031621 (ebook) | ISBN 9781032217062 (paperback) | ISBN 9781032217055 (hardback) | ISBN 9781003269649 (ebook)
Subjects: LCSH: Psychic trauma--Social aspects. | Psychoanalysis--Social aspects.
Classification: LCC BF175.5.P75 P79 2023 (print) | LCC BF175.5.P75 (ebook) | DDC 155.9/3--dc23/eng/20220921
LC record available at https://lccn.loc.gov/2022031620
LC ebook record available at https://lccn.loc.gov/2022031621

ISBN: 978-1-032-21705-5 (hbk)
ISBN: 978-1-032-21706-2 (pbk)
ISBN: 978-1-003-26964-9 (ebk)

DOI: 10.4324/9781003269649

Typeset in Times New Roman
by KnowledgeWorks Global Ltd.

Contents

Contributors

Klimis Navridis was born in Athens, Greece, and is a Professor Emeritus of Psychology of the Psychology Faculty of the National and Kapodistrian University of Athens. He also works as a psychoanalyst and group psychotherapist. He is a member of the Hellenic Society of Psychoanalytic Psychotherapy, of the French Association of Psychoanalytic Group Psychotherapy (SFPPG) and founding member, training and supervising group analyst and president of the Hellenic Society for Psychoanalytic Group Psychotherapy (HSPGP). He has published more than 60 papers in international scientific journals. He is the author of several books: *Alice in the Objects-land: The Child as Advertising Object* (1986), *Clinical Social Psychology* (1994), *Group Psychology: A Clinical Psychodynamic Approach* (2005) and *Groupishness and Mediation* (2011). He was visiting Professor at the Universities of Louvain-La-Neuve (Belgium), Angers UC (France) and Paris VII and Editor-in-Chief of the scientific revue "Psychology" of the Hellenic Psychological Society (2001–2006). He has also been President of the Hellenic Psychological Society (2006–2013) and President of the Pedagogical Institute of Greece (2010–2012).

Wojtek Hanbowski is a psychoanalyst, member of the Polish Psychoanalytical Society and Hana Segal Institute for Psychoanalytical Studies. In the 1990s, he had his psychoanalytical training in London where he also worked at the Cassel Hospital and Parkside Clinic.

Daniela Lucarelli is a psychologist, psychoanalyst, and full member at the IPA/SPI and an IPA recognised expert on children and adolescents. She is co-chair of the IPA Couple and Family Committee and Editor-in-Chief of the IACFP Review (Review of the International Association Couple and Family Psychoanalysis). Daniela is a teacher and supervisor at Istituto Winnicott in Rome, founding member of SIPsIA (*Società Italiana di Psicoterapia Psicoanalitica dell'Infanzia e dell'Adolescenza e della Coppia*) in Rome, and teacher and supervisor at PCF (*Corso*

Postspecialistico di Psicoanalisi della Coppia e della Famiglia) in Rome. She is a member of the editorial board of Interazioni (Franco Angeli, Milan) and author of publications on children, adolescents and couple and family psychoanalysis.

Gianluca Biggio is Professor of Organizational Psychology and Communication, senior member with training function and past Scientific Coordinator of SIPP (Italian Society of Psychoanalytic Psychotherapy), senior member of EFPP (European Psychoanalytic Psychotherapy for the public Sector) and member of EAWOP (European Association of Organizational and Work Psychology). He has published scientific articles and books at the national and international level on psychoanalytic psychotherapy, counselling and organizational psychology. He has held scientific responsibility for various European projects (on elderly assistance in 2012–2014; on prison health barriers in 2013–2015; on restorative justice in 2021–2023). He was Visiting Professor in the psychology departments in Norway, Spain, Portugal, Canada, Australia and Scotland.

Morris Nitsun is a consultant clinical psychologist, psychotherapist, and group analyst. He is a member of the Fitzrovia Group Analytic Practice and a training analyst at the Institute of Group Analysis, London. He retired in 2020 from the UK National Health Service in which he was head of psychology and psychotherapy for 30 years. He is a widely published author whose books, *The Anti-Group: Destructive Forces in the Group and Their Creative Potential* and *The Group as an Object of Desire* have been described as "classics in the field." He has lectured extensively in the UK and abroad. He is also a practising artist whose new book, *A Psychotherapist Paints*, is due for publication in 2022.

Lida Anagnostaki, MSc, PhD, is an Associate Professor in Psychodynamic Perspectives in Developmental Psychology, Department of Early Childhood Education, National and Kapodistrian University of Athens and a full member of the Hellenic Association of Child and Adolescent Psychoanalytic Psychotherapy. Her research interests include parent-child separation, psychoanalysis and education, and psychoanalytically informed research.

Alexandra Zaharia, MD, is a child psychiatrist and a child and adolescent psychoanalytic psychotherapist, and full member and member of the Supervisors' Committee of the Hellenic Association of Child and Adolescent Psychoanalytic Psychotherapy. Her research interests include the setting in the child and adolescent psychoanalytic psychotherapy, trauma and parent-child separation.

Vladimir Jović, MD, DMSci (Doctor of Medical Science), is a psychiatrist, psychoanalyst and a training analyst of the Belgrade Psychoanalytic

Society (BPS) and former President of the BPS (2014–2018). He works in psychiatric and psychoanalytical private practice in Belgrade. He is one of the founders and currently a consultant of the Center for Rehabilitation of Torture Victims, IAN, Belgrade, which is providing comprehensive rehabilitation for victims and implementing activities on the prevention of torture in Serbia and the region. Since September 2020, he has been a member of the board of trustees of the United Nations Voluntary Fund for Victims of Torture. His primary research area is psychological trauma and psychosocial mechanisms of violence and torture.

Sverre Varvin, MD, Doctor of Philosophy, is training in the Norwegian Psychoanalytic Society and Professor Emeritus at Oslo Metropolitan University. He has worked clinically and done research on traumatization and treatment of traumatized patients, especially in the refugee field. He has conducted process and outcome research on psychoanalytic therapy, research on traumatic dreams and on psychoanalytic training. He has twice been president of the Norwegian Psychoanalytic Society and has had several positions in the IPA, including his present role as chair of the IPA China Committee. He has published articles and books on traumatization, refugees, terrorism and on research on treatment process and outcome.

Teresa von Sommaruga Howard is the daughter of a German Jewish refugee father and non-Jewish British mother. Born in England, she grew up in Aotearoa, New Zealand but now lives in the UK and works internationally. Teresa's professional background mirrors her diverse personal background. She is an architect, systemic family therapist and group analyst, mainly focusing on the long-term effects of socio-political trauma mainly through working with larger groups in many settings around the world. This focus led her to set up a unique series of connected workshops, "Creating Large Group Dialogue in Organisations and Society" in 2019, which has since flourished with many international members. She has written and published extensively about all aspects of her work and co-authored a book, *Design through Dialogue: A Guide for Clients and Architects* (Wiley, 2010), which integrates her background as both an architect and group analyst. She is also co-editor of *The Journey Home: Emerging Out of the Shadow of the Past* (Peter Lang, 2022), an anthology that brings together 20 contributions with commentary about the transgenerational effects of catastrophic trauma.

Ludovica Grassi is a child neuro-psychiatrist and a full member of the Italian Society of Psychoanalysis, IPA and EFPP. She is a qualified expert in child and adolescent psychoanalysis, and a psychoanalyst of couples and families. She is currently Treasurer of the Italian Psychoanalytic Society. Her book *The Sound of the Unconscious: Psychoanalysis as Music* was published by Routledge in June 2021.

Eftychia-Evie Athanassiadou, PhD, MSc, is a clinical psychologist and psychotherapist of children and adolescents. She is member of the Hellenic Association of Child and Adolescent Psychoanalytic Psychotherapy and has been working for the last 20 years in mental health units for children and adolescents as a psychotherapist, clinical manager and presently as supervisor ("Aghia Sophia" Children's Hospital Child Psychiatric Clinic, University of Athens Medical School, APHCA). She has taught in graduate and postgraduate programs in collaboration with East London University and the University of Athens Department of Clinical Psychology. For many years, she was an instructor of infant observation in the program of HACAPP and in other university programs on the mental health of infants and toddlers. At this stage, she works privately in Athens but also as a psychotherapy and clinical supervisor in public and private day centers for traumatized children and adolescents.

Tija Despotovic, MD, is a psychiatrist, psychoanalyst and group analyst, and has worked at the Psychiatric Clinic, University Clinical Centre Serbia. She is currently in private psychotherapeutic practice with individuals and groups. She has been a training analyst for the Belgrade Psychoanalytic Society IPA, the Association of Individual Psychoanalytic Psychotherapists, a training group analyst for GASB, one of the founders and former Chair of Group Analytic Society Belgrade (GASB), Chair of the GA Training in GASB and involved in Group Analytic Training in India. Tija is a EGATIN Committee member, GASI MC member and former GASI Summer School Chair. She has written papers on psychic pain, mourning, social trauma and psychotherapy with difficult patients.

Mary Morgan is a psychoanalyst and couple psychoanalytic psychotherapist. She is a Fellow of the British Psychoanalytic Society, Senior Fellow of Tavistock Relationships, Honorary Member of the Polish Psychoanalytic Society and Consultant to the IPA Committee of Couple and Family Psychoanalysis. She has contributed many key articles and chapters in the field of couple psychoanalysis and her recent book is *A Couple State of Mind: Couple Psychoanalysis and the Tavistock Relationships Model.* She teaches and supervises internationally and has a private psychoanalytic practice.

Gila Ofer, PhD, is clinical psychologist, training psychoanalyst and group analyst. Dr. Ofer is the founder and past president of the Tel-Aviv Institute of Contemporary Psychoanalysis (TAICP) and a founding member of the Israeli Institute of Group Analysis (IIGA) and she serves on the faculty of both institutes and at the Post-Graduate School for Psychoanalytic Psychotherapy, Tel-Aviv University. Dr. Ofer has been the chair of the group analytic section and board member of the EFPP, and later a conjoint member of the board as the coordinator of Eastern European countries of the EFPP. Currently she is the editor of the *EFPP Psychoanalytic Psychotherapy Review.* She has published her work in leading journals and presented her work and taught in Israel, Europe, East Asia and the United States. Her edited book, *A Bridge over Troubled Water: Conflicts and Reconciliation in Group and Society*, was published in 2017.

Bojana Mitrović is a psychologist, psychotherapist, group analyst and member of the Group Analytic Society Belgrade and Group Analytic Society International. Bojana works in private practice as a psychotherapist, as well as for a research company in media research. She lives and works in Belgrade.

Snežana Kecojević Miljević, MD, is a psychiatrist, psychoanalytic psychotherapist, supervisor and training group analyst, currently in the private sector in Belgrade. She is president of the Association of Psychoanalytic Psychotherapists of Serbia, member of the Training Committee of Group Analytic Society Belgrade, member of the Presidency of Serbian Medical Society and Serbian delegate for Adult Section EFFP.

Vida Rakić Glišić, MD, MS, is a psychiatrist, training group analyst and psychoanalyst. She is co-founder of the Group Analytic Society Belgrade (GASB), Belgrade Psychoanalytic Society (BPS) and the Society for Children and Adolescent Psychotherapy. She is a member of the Society of Serbian Doctors, Society for Psychoanalytic Psychotherapy, GASB, BPS, the Group Analytic Society International (GASI) and the International Psychoanalytic Association (IPA). She works in private practice with children, adolescents, adults and various groups. Vida enjoys clinical work, teaching, supervising and writing, and is presently serving the fifth year as the president of the Ethics Committee of DGAB. For many years, she has been acting as a referee of the *Group Analysis Journal*, The International Journal of Group-Analytic Psychotherapy, SAGE, London.

Jelica Satarić, MD, is a psychiatrist, individual psychotherapist, and group analyst in private practice in Belgrade. She is member of the Serbian Medical Chamber, the Serbian Psychiatric Association and the Group Analytic Society Belgrade (GAS-Belgrade), of which she is the president, and a training group analyst. She is a member of Group Analytic Society International (GASI).

Or Netanely is a clinical psychologist and an executive coach in private practice in Tel Aviv. Since 2014, he and his co-authors have been interested in community dreaming gatherings, to explore the unconscious underpinnings of the torn Israeli society and help communities to know themselves and heal.

Hanni Biran is a clinical psychologist, training psychoanalyst, member of the Tel Aviv Institute of Contemporary Psychoanalysis, as well as a group analyst and a member of the Israeli Institute for Group Analysis.

Judith Ezra is a social worker, group analyst, and staff member at Bar Ilan University. In her private practice, she works with individuals, couples, families and groups. She has a philosophy degree and she is researching and writing about links and connections between psychoanalysis and Kabbalah.

Hanan Sabah Teicher is a clinical psychologist and one of the founders of "Mekomi," a therapist cooperative in Tel Aviv.

Ivanka Dunjić, MD, is a psychiatrist, psychoanalyst and group analyst in private practice in Belgrade. She is a founding member and former chair of Belgrade Group Analytic Society (DGAB), founding member and former chair of training in the Belgrade Psychoanalytic Society (BPD), former chair of Serbian Society for Psychoanalytic Psychotherapy (DPPS), member of GAI (Group Analysis India) faculty, a teaching and supervising analyst and group analyst in Belgrade.

Giuliana Marin is a psychologist-psychotherapist with a psychoanalytic orientation who works with children, adolescents, parental couples and families. She is a couple and family psychotherapist of the PCF, the Italian Society of Couple and Family Psychoanalysis, and is a member of the EFPP and AIPCF (International Association of Couple and Family Psychoanalysis) and a consultant psychologist and psychotherapist at the Rittmeyer Regional Institute for the Blind in Trieste, where she deals mainly with children, adolescents of couples and families. She is a former Honorary Judge of the Court of Minors of Trieste and former teacher in the School of Specialization "Life Cycle Psychology" and "Neuropsychology" of Trieste on youth problems and in various training courses related to parenting.

Mariagrazia Giachin is a psychoanalytic psychotherapist of the Psychoanalysis Italian Society of Couple and Family (PCF), member of AIPCF (International Association of Couple and Family Psychoanalysis) and is currently attending the "PANDEMIA Group" — Study Center, Scientific Center — AIPCF. Mariagrazia has been a psychologist/psychotherapist for 30 years in the National Health Service dealing with the life cycle of the family, focusing in particular on the issues of adoption and abuse and the mistreatment of children. She was a supervisor of Antiviolence Centers and Shelter Homes from 2013 to 2021, a teacher at Health and Social Assistance Service operators and an Adjunct Professor at the University of Trieste. She is an author of articles on the topic of clinical activity.

Introduction

Anna Maria Nicolò

This book deals with a theme that is becoming more and more central to the understanding of individual psychology and also of group and social functioning. COVID pandemics, wars and genocides are phenomena that are disrupting the world, including our Western societies. The relevant feature of this publication is to compare analysts of different nationalities, using different settings, but all working on the field of trauma.

It revolves around four crucial themes: the analysis of trauma and its post-traumatic effects; work in individual, couple and group settings; and reflections on the political and social aspects of collective trauma and on the instruments for its elaboration, such as cinema. It will not be possible for me in this introduction to testify to the richness of the various chapters or even to quote them all, but reading them has enriched me and made me reflect.

In the course of time, we have experienced traumas such as genocides and migrations that have affected history, caused by man's violent action on man. Unfortunately, even if we must admit that—as Horace said—"*Nihil humanum a me alienum puto*" (there is nothing about human events that I feel is strained and different from me), it seems to us with amazement that the final product of such traumas is dehumanization. Primo Levi, in his book titled, *If This is a Man*, refers to this because it questions the extent to which violence, torture, and sadism are capable of stripping individuals of the characteristics that create humanity. Yet, as a demonstration of man's creative capacities, an impressive theoretical reflection has originated from these experiences. Just think of the discoveries on the themes of loss and separation in the development of personality, the studies on the effects of trauma, and dozens of psychoanalytic societies have been founded as a result of these events.

Indeed, we can say, as Klimis Navridis states, that "The traumatic, has been the cornerstone of psychoanalysis." I will only recall that, during the Second World War, Anna Freud founded the Hampstead War Nurseries, a home for more than 100 children wounded in the war, and that British psychoanalyst Donald Winnicott's work had very important social effects,

DOI: 10.4324/9781003269649-1

allowing in 1948 the production of the "Children Act," an Act of Parliament that established the childcare service in Great Britain.

This book is a striking demonstration of this by showing with great accuracy in-depth reflections around what trauma produces in the internal world of individuals and how it affects external realities. The chapter by Sverre Varvin, Tija Despotovic and Vladimir Jović on the Psychotherapy of Post-traumatic Conditions illustrates with great precision and depth the effects of traumatic experiences in their destructive impact on the capacity for symbolization and affect regulation.

The great risk of these traumatisms is the fact that they do not end in the here and now, but enter the transgenerational chain of transmission of memory, which, as we know, consists in a crossing, between generations, between psychic spaces, of contents whose elaboration and transformation has not been possible. Some of the authors of this book examine them, such as Mariagrazia Giachin and Giuliana Marin, who highlight the role of family myth in this regard.

Yolanda Gampel (2000) recalls the effect of overpowering stimuli, in the psychic apparatus when our perceptual and representational systems become loaded with "the representational leftover that permeate through themselves the transgenerational transmission."

Ferenczi (2018) spoke in this regard of "dead clinical fragments, exiled parts of the mind from the conscious and unconscious [which] can, that is, appear through other languages," through the somatic route for example, as we have seen in many cases, that inscription in the body which represents one of the vehicles of the most primitive communication. But even everyday actions can be an expressive language that is constructed in the everyday life in the group, especially in family groups, which becomes an organizational modality of the traumatic links that are transmitted from parent to child in successive generations and that we can observe in family myths or in the myths of a people.

Traumas then determine a particular type of memories, preserved in a totally different way than autobiographical memory (Van der Kolk et al., 1996). They are perpetuated in a timeless dimension that is neither "modified nor reshaped by subjective meaning, cognitive schemas, or unconscious expectations or phantasies" (Bohleber, 2007).

Varvin recalls how the traumatized patient from the beginning of therapy will engage the analyst in a non-symbolized, unconscious, usually acted out relationship through which patient communicates his or her traumatic experiences (Varvin, 2013). Varvin, Despotovic and Jovic dwell on a clinical theme of enormous importance and topicality, that of enactment considered by these authors as "a collapse in the therapeutic dialogue in which the analyst is involved in an interaction in which he acts unconsciously, thus actualizing the unconscious desires of both himself and the patient."

This is another of the enriching effects that trauma studies have produced, highlighting the deep communications that traumatic experiences inscribed in the unremoved unconscious produce in the interaction between analyst and patient. This opens the way not only to a deeper understanding in the analytic couple, but also to a starting point for a radical change in technique and therapeutic goals, no longer based only on the unveiling of the unconscious, but rather on the creation of new experiences or on giving form and symbolization to formless experiences, such as those present in the primitive states of the mind.

The suffering resulting from these traumas will then be at the center of a crucible amid the intrapsychic, the interpersonal and the transpersonal, that is the psyche of the individual, that of the group to which he belongs such as the family and the institution where he works and society, as Sigmund Freud himself pointed out about the psychology of the masses and as Gila Ofer highlights in his work. For Ofer, during the COVID pandemic, one of the current traumas that has characterized our time, important ethical and technical dilemmas were highlighted, since some dramatic problems of our world were clearly seen, such as those produced by a system of ruthless capitalization or social disparity between rich and poor, old and young. For Gianluca Biggio, the globalization of technology and migration processes appears in the responses of the groups. Other studies address the theme of the group in the analysis such as Jelica Satarić, Bojana Mitrović, Teresa von Sommaruga Howard, or even Morris Nitsun. Ulrich Schultz-Venrath shows us a group psychotherapy based on mentalization. Interesting then is the experience made during the national congress of Serbian psychotherapists of working on a large group, as Snezana Kecojević Miljević, Vida Rakić Glišić and Satarić show us.

A part of these works is dedicated to the collective trauma produced by the pandemic. In many nations of the world, psychotherapists have been forced to modify the setting in an attempt to help their patients cope with the terrible consequences of this trauma. Many observations have resulted. In this book, Eftychia-Evie Athanassiadou studies the effect of the absence of the therapist's body in the setting with the child and adolescent. Mary Morgan examines individual and couple patients' experiences of the analytic process during the COVID pandemic. In some of these couples, increased intimacy was observed while in others, a claustrophobic situation was highlighted compromising "the couple's mental state." This notation is the element that characterizes the work with the couple and the family as it is also made explicit by all the studies on the bond as a third element, co-constructed by the members in interaction (Berenstein & Puget, 2008; Pichon-Rivière, 1980; Nicolò, 2014).

On another side, Cristina Călărășanu shows the power and effectiveness of a widely used social tool like cinema. She states, "Romanian cinema was the chosen medium after the fall of communism to elaborate and symbolize some of the traces of social traumata" and in fact cinema is "a symbolic tool that puts images and words where there was a blank." In this way, a history of social trauma is also written that does not close its eyes to the unhealed wounds that remain as a social legacy of it. It is indeed important not to consciously forget this history, even if oblivion, memory and the vicissitudes of memory are the axes on which the necessary psychic work is articulated.

Part of the book is dedicated to the consequences of migration, a phenomenon that has strongly characterized the last 40 years. Daniela Lucarelli and Ludovica Grassi examine how adolescence and migration can unleash ancient transgenerational traumas that weigh on the family and the individual, initiating a renegotiation of the original narcissistic contract. Problems of integration, assimilation, because of this can emerge in the first as well as in the second and third generation. In the original work of Lida Anagnostaki and Alexandra Zaharia, the effect of migration is observed in those who, instead of leaving, remain in the country of origin, showing how these children, "little Telemachus," are affected by the early and prolonged separation from their parents, as happened to the son of Ulysses, Telemachus.

The message of this collective work, however, emerges as strong and significant, and is also an expression of the sensitivity and attention that the European Federation of Psychoanalytic Psychotherapy has toward a central theme of psychoanalysis and of our times. Today, the collective trauma is imposed in all its raw reality, it is a fact even before being an experience and the mind can be overwhelmed. External reality has become prevalent, it has crossed the boundaries of the self, of the person, and has imposed itself in all its concreteness.

In this sense, this book, even though it studies the work in the consultation room (Ivanka Dunjić), even before observing the articulation between the mental functioning of the individual and the trauma, shows that, in order to understand the phenomenon, we need to articulate the individual psyche and the collective psyche, which are functioning that respond to quite different rules, both in their effects and in the defenses they activate.

The question remains alive as to whether psychoanalysis as a method can intervene by offering help or instead, when faced with phenomena of a social and collective nature that touch on areas of the unconscious that Kaës (2016) defines as ectopic and extrapsychic, it must step back and respectfully retreat, appealing only to what Freud called the work of culture (*Kulturarbeit*).

Psychoanalytic research in recent years has investigated some possible applications of the psychoanalytic method to other settings. While up to 20 years ago these applications (or, as we say today, extensions of the method) caused rejection or conflict at least at the institutional level, today many people study and write about them, where at the beginning they expressed open criticism. This book, and in particular some of its chapters, show how the psychoanalytic approach can offer a specific tool to deal on a technical level with the effects of collective trauma beyond what can take place in the classical setting.

However, there are some invariants that characterize the method in any setting and they consist, in my opinion, on the one hand in the construction of a possible setting, on the other hand in what I would call an "elaborative listening," a listening that looks not only at the word of the other, at the discourse, to fantasies and dreams, but also to actions, somatizations, our own and the other's sensations, to the unconscious in its different manifestations of repressed and non-repressed unconscious, to all the ways in which archaic experiences reactivated by the massiveness of the current trauma are expressed in the urgency.

In these situations, the particular presence of the analyst as a multi-level witness, in the interpersonal encounter, of the dramatic event in reality, which he or she shares, is crucial. This can alleviate pain by counteracting the defensive processes that lead to rejection, denial and forgetting. The analyst's testimony also has a meaning with respect to the social pact because it means being able to resume trust in the other, in listening to the other, in the recognition of existence that the other can give you. Freud (1950[1895]) had stated that the psychoanalyst is called to be the *Nebenmensch*, the close human being. The Nebenmensch is the person who listens properly to the call of the child but, above all, is the interlocutor who accompanies in the acquisition of speech. The Nebenmensch is not, however, a passive witness precisely because we are actually speaking for the analyst of an active, participatory position, and this experience involves him on many levels, starting with his somatic counter-transference.

Today, psychoanalysis meets with enormous cultural and social changes and with the very changes in the pathology of our patients, and all these works show the importance of psychoanalysis in responding to the deep needs in society. Needs that are not processed today risk turning into serious psychopathological problems tomorrow.

To give a wide and at the same time deep presence, psychoanalysis must make a complex operation: on the one hand we must precisely define the invariants of our method, but at the same time be able to modify some aspects of the technique to be effective in different settings. This has already happened in the past where our clinic has encountered different ages of life or different pathologies, i.e. with children and adolescents but also with psychotic and borderline patients.

It is now necessary to study carefully how to contribute to the cure even when dealing with collective traumas such as emigration or pandemics or wars. The transformation of the other is always ours as well.

References

Berenstein I., Puget J., Psychanalyse du Lien. Ed. Erès, Paris, 2008.

Bohleber W., Remémoration, traumatisme et mémoire collective. Le combat pour la remémoration psychanalyse. Revue française de psychanalyse, 71(3):803–830, 2007.

Ferenczi S., Psicoanalisi delle nevrosi di guerra. In: Fondamenti di psicoanalisi, vol. III, Guaraldi Editore, Rimini, 2018.

Freud S., Project for a Scientific Psychology (1950 [1895]). The Standard Edition of the Complete Psychological Works of Sigmund Freud, Volume I (1886-1899): Pre-Psycho-Analytic Publications and Unpublished Drafts, pp. 281–391, 1950.

Gampel Y., Io sono (il feroce e trionfante) re del castello. Richard e Piggle, 8(2):191–202, 2000.

Kaës R., L'estensione della psicoanalisi, FrancoAngeli, Milano, 2016.

Levi P., Se questo è un uomo, Torino: F. De Silva, coll. "Biblioteca Leone Ginzburg" n. 3, 1947.

Nicolò A.M., Where is the unconscious located? Reflection on links in families and couples. In: Nicolò A.M., Benghozi P., Lucarelli D. (eds). Families in Transformations, Karnac, London, 2014.

Pichon-Rivière E., Teoria del vinculo, Nueva Vision, Buenos Aires, 1980.

Van der Kolk B.A., McFarlane A.C., Weisaeth L, Traumatic Stress: The Effects of Overwhelming Experience on Mind, Body and Society, Guilford Press, New York, 1996.

Varvin S. e Volkan V.D., (a cura di). Violenza o dialogo. Insight psicoanalitico su terrore e terrorismo, Edizioni Borla, Roma, 2006.

Part I

Trauma Stories and History

Chapter 1

Finding My Song

Trauma, Discontinuity and the Large Group

Teresa von Sommaruga Howard

We were standing, looking up at the huge steel Mahnmal Levetzowstrasse, the memorial to the Transports to Auschwitz from Berlin, when my father suddenly said, "I have just realised something. If I had not left when I did, I would not be here now. Neither would you. It's quite a thought isn't it!"

Not only was he no longer living in the city where he had grown up, but before this moment, he had not been able to imagine what might have happened to him if he had not left as a lone 15-year-old refugee in 1936. Later, he was interned by the British government as an Enemy Alien in June 1940 (Lafitte, 1940 & 1988). When the war was over, and to get as far away as possible from Europe, we emigrated as a family to Aotearoa, New Zealand.

Growing up, I knew the bones of this history, but I had no idea what it meant. German, Jew, Enemy Alien, Internment, Dunera and Berlin were all words I heard, but I could never fully grasp their impact. It is significant that I never heard 'deportation' to describe what actually happened to my father when he was shipped to Australia on the 'Dunera.' That was the one experience he could never talk about. It was while writing this chapter that this word deportation presented itself. What I grew up with was the feeling that something powerful had happened. I had little idea what it was, but it had an emotional force of radioactive intensity that we could all feel but never find words for. It wasn't until he was in his 90s that he told me over the breakfast table, "I know it's stupid, but I feel such shame for not being able to stop what happened to me and the others." He was talking about being interned by the British as an Enemy Alien. After he died, I discovered his diaries and many letters written to newspapers and politicians, all in pencil on anything he could find, including toilet paper. He was 19.

Trauma had prevented my dad from recognising the cost of his survival and the torment of the first 21 years of his life. To protect himself from remembering too much, he had cut himself off from family and friends and moved as far away from the source of his life-threatening experiences as he could. His solution was reinforced by the cultural mores of the post-war period. As Aleida Assmann, Professor of Literature at the University of

DOI: 10.4324/9781003269649-3

Konstanz, explains, "in the aftermath of wars, a collective forgetting was decreed so as to neutralize memories that could endanger the peaceful coexistence of the victors and the defeated" (Assmann, 2016: 92). When the present is disconnected from the past, the twin mechanisms of not only forgetting but also removing all reminders of a life lost provide the first generation with relief from horror. For the next generation, it means living in an empty space between past and present with a history that cannot be told.

To illustrate, although I grew up knowing there was such a thing as Pesach that is celebrated with a Seder, the ritual meal that tells the story of coming out of Egypt, I had never experienced it or learnt to cook the special food until quite late in life.

After the ritual telling of the story, the meal traditionally starts with matzo ball soup. Matzo balls are small dumplings made with a special flour that does not rise. It is used for this festival to remember the quick exit from Egypt. I had made this soup many times using different recipes, but my matzo balls were either like little rocks or slushy. This year when I arrived at my friend's kitchen, the preparation was still in progress. She asked me to help roll the matzo balls. I looked at the mixture in the bowl: a sloppy mess. How on earth does one roll this into balls? I noticed the bowl of cold water nearby. "Dip your hands in the water. It is important that they are moist!" Presto! It was possible to roll the sloppy mixture into balls.

This was the first time someone had shown me how. My father loved them but could never show me how they were made. My effort to bridge this discontinuity alone had only been partially successful. It needed someone from my father's lost culture to demonstrate. It is this discontinuity and its wider societal implications that I intend exploring in this paper.

Discontinuity and Rupture

Working to understand my family history alerted me to a feeling of being suspended between an unknown past and a disconnected present: at home nowhere. Despite my dad's protestations that Aotearoa, New Zealand, was the best place in the world, he had to work hard to feel at home in a culture where few people could comprehend his background. He constantly struggled to make sense of his longing for a country that had expelled him. When he was invited back to Berlin just after his 80th birthday, he made an impassioned speech at a reception in the German Bundestag about how the European Union (EU) had put a wall around Europe that allowed nothing in. "They think they are the centre of the universe, but Asia and the Pacific are where it's at." Now almost 20 years later, I realise that he was also telling the Germans how painful it still was to have been forced to leave his birth country. Thinking about this event much later, I realised that he was giving voice to a deeply buried humiliation that he took with him to his grave.

What happened to my father happened to thousands, perhaps millions, of others. They suffered the destruction of a complete social context that took apart their whole community, culture and way of life. Everything familiar and known disappeared. Those who, as I write, take the perilous journey to Europe and across Europe to try to find a safer place to live suffer the same dilemma.

Having fled, refugees discover that the host culture is not only quite uninterested in their heritage, but more significantly, deeply resents and works hard to repel them. A recent collection of visual and written essays, *The System of Systems*, shows how political powers in Europe use bureaucratic systems to keep asylum seekers out (Glyn-Blanco, McLintock, & Papazymouri, 2017). This book contains a map of Europe superimposed with concentric rings, a bit like the zones on a city transport map. The inner zone includes the states of northwestern Europe: France, Britain, Germany and Scandinavia; the middle zone, countries on the southern and eastern edge of EU, including Spain, Italy, Greece, Bulgaria, Slovakia and Poland; and the outer zone, countries immediately outside the EU, including Turkey, North African states and Ukraine.

There is a myth in Britain that refugees from Hitler were proudly welcomed. It is quite untrue. Not only do I have my father's experience to inform me, but I came across a report from two academics at the University of East Anglia to the All-Party Parliamentary Group on Archives and History, *Refugee History: the 1930s crisis and today* (Taylor & Ferguson, 2017). Those who did make it into the country did so thanks to the work of civil organisations and volunteers. It is chilling to learn how Britain shirked its responsibilities not simply by building walls, but with the far stronger barricades of mean-minded administrative procedures (ibid, 2017: 4). Commenting on this report in the New Statesman, Julia Rampen suggests that Britain's treatment of refugees fleeing the Nazis is a story of brutality cloaked in bureaucracy. Of an estimated 500,000 to 600,000 family and individual case files showing efforts to bring refugees to Britain before the Second World War, only an estimated 80,000 were successful and came with the understanding that they would emigrate as soon as possible to a third country: a success rate of just 16 percent (Rampen, 2018). Louise London, a solicitor who has dealt with modern-day refugees (and is herself the child of Jewish refugees) draws attention to treasury records that demonstrate that even in 1933 "British policy towards the refugees revolved around the issue of finance." It was only after the Anglo-Jewish community promised that any Jewish refugee admitted would not become a burden on the state that the government decided not to introduce further restrictions on German Jews seeking to enter Britain (London, 2001: 26). Nothing changes. The recent Windrush scandal and the Brexit decision illustrate the same desire to "Keep all those 'bloody' foreigners out!"

Quite apart from the desire to maintain physical exclusion, there is another much more subtle form of exclusion at work: the tendency to exclude the reality of a newcomer's suffering from any conversation. Elie Wiesel, in the second edition of his book, *Night*, describes this dilemma very well:

> Deep down, the witness knew then, as he does now, that his testimony would not be received. After all, it deals with an event that sprang from the darkest zone of man. Only those who experienced Auschwitz know what it was. Others will never know.
>
> But would they at least understand?
>
> (Wiesel, 2006: ix)

Although dramatic, it explains how difficult it is not only to tell about horrific experiences but also how difficult it is for others to hear about them. Without the possibility to tell, individual memory remains just that, an isolated individual memory. Without witnesses who can listen, the memory cannot be connected with the memories of others to be enriched and confirmed and renders the experience invisible.

Looking for 'Home': A Driving Force

To escape the threat of physical annihilation, refugees are forced to find refuge in a new country becoming physically and emotionally homeless, losing their class status along the way. Professional dreams are no longer possible. They become servants, no longer having servants themselves and usually end up living in the poorest areas of the new country. Everything that was familiar and could be relied upon disappears, creating a rupture in the continuity of culture and context, of friends and places. Nothing is as it was, and nothing can be taken for granted. Even when the spoken language is apparently the same, cultural clues are different. Nothing and nowhere feels like home.

As well as the obvious physical dislocation, there is an often-unrecognised emotional dislocation. Without appropriate mirroring or cultural resonance, wounds remain invisible and little if any healing can occur. Immigrants are constantly reminded that there is something unacceptable about their reactions, feelings and thoughts in this new place. This is a form of racism, even terrorisation, that insists newcomers fit in and forget their origins. As Dalal suggests, "Black people born in Britain do not belong to the British 'us,' which is made identical to whiteness, but to a different category Black British, which is 'not us'" (2002: 205).

To survive, refugees focus their energies on picking up what pieces are left and building a new future, but their dreams are inevitably limited by the new context. Host countries do not want them, are not interested in who they are or where they came from and expect them to integrate or assimilate quickly. The pressure is to 'move on' or 'let go'." The central defining experience of newcomers' lives is ignored. Hannah Arendt (1943) writes about how the Jews who came to the United Kingdom (UK) in the 1930s as refugees strained every sinew to fit in, to become invisible, to be the best newcomers they could possibly be: "We wanted to rebuild our lives, that was all. In order to rebuild one's life one has to be strong and an optimist. So, we are very optimistic."

The next generation has no memories of the 'old country' but they know two things: their parents' longing and the reality of the present. Without the experience of their origins, the inevitable confusion makes it very difficult to make sense of their own history and identity. Always feeling like a misfit, it is not easy to resist the pull to fit in.

Growing up in New Zealand, I lived with the prevailing socio-political assumption that everybody was Christian. I still experience it as alienating while there. I remember the 1956 Israeli war. I was only 13 then. Feeling my father's panic, I felt impelled to drop everything to join the fight against those 'marauding' Arabs. Reflecting now on this reactive response, I had no real idea that I was looking for a home, but it gives me a clue now about why apparently well-settled and UK-born Muslim youngsters decide to travel to Syria or Iraq or elsewhere to fight with ISIS or to become suicide bombers in European cities.

Why Suicide Bombers?

Just as it was for me growing up in New Zealand, the next generation from the Middle East living in Europe is suspended between two cultures. However, there is a significant difference between these two experiences. Europe is in the middle of a cultural war with the Middle East. Alongside this overt animosity between their country of origin and country of refuge, they live with their parents' longing and their own confusion. As a young Syrian refugee recently told me, she finds her mind in constant oscillation between exile and refuge. Nowhere feels like home. This is not only personal but also political. Living in a Western materialist culture full of animosity toward Islam while her home country is being bombed out of existence makes it almost impossible to settle. She watches helplessly, worrying about friends and family as the physical and social infrastructure that connects them to their history, culture and identity is being systematically destroyed. It is the same suspended experience of never feeling at home I described at the beginning of this paper.

Realpolitik has left a terrible legacy in the Middle East. It is often forgotten what the West has done with its political meddling and imperialist ambitions. The war between Iran and Iraq is a case in point. According to Simon Tisdall, writing in the Guardian about current American policy toward Iran, "the Iranian People's real offence was their presumptuous overthrow of the Shah's autocratic, pro-American regime in the 1979 revolution." He suggests this was the genesis of the lethal US backing for Saddam Hussein in the 1980–88 Iran-Iraq war that took 300,000 Iranian lives. It was a national trauma, yet there has been no US apology (Tisdall, 2018). When the balance of power becomes so asymmetrical, Ami Pedahzur, an Israeli Academic, suggests that weaker states use whatever means they have at their disposal to fight for their position. Suicide campaigns are employed as a political strategy when there is no other hope of being taken seriously enough for dialogue to begin (Pedahzur, 2005).

But how do regimes encourage people to tie a suicide belt around their waist or to get into a vehicle packed with explosives?

In Iran, Ayatollah Ruhollah Khomeini needed popular support for sending young children to die on the battlefield and so he used his religious authority to ensure suicide could be seen a praiseworthy act of self-sacrifice (*istishhad* in Arabic) (Pedahzur, 2005: 161). He used his religious authority to encourage a 'culture of death' in which the idea of joining the army and becoming a hero, even a martyr, was spread among boys in Iran. What started as top-down propaganda was translated into peer pressure, a mechanism not unlike that depicted in the film, *All Quiet on the Western Front*, for recruiting schoolboys to fight in the First World War. Other countries in the area and groups such as Hezbollah, struggling to make their voices heard, did not need much convincing—posters of *shahids* (martyrs) became a cultural icon for Palestinians. Suicide death became a way of restoring pride and self-esteem.

Having established a culture that applauds suicide death, it does not take much to recognise that vulnerable young kids with a need to belong can easily be encouraged to act as human bombs. Unacknowledged dislocating experiences make one vulnerable to being volunteered or volunteering for "nationalist" crusades when there is a promise of finding a home, perhaps for the first time. In the Islamic diaspora, promises of a new version of the old culture are used to seduce the children of refugees to fight for a new utopia in this way. Remembering what my father said about the shame he had no reason to feel, I also wonder about how a wish to exorcise the humiliating experience of being a refugee family contributes to the decision to sacrifice oneself in this way.

The Larger Group as a Place of Repair

What I have been describing is a form of social trauma and yet, according to Patrick Bracken, a British psychiatrist with experience working with victims of torture, it is this social aspect that has been systematically sidelined. Instead, a strongly individualistic focus that presents trauma as something that happens inside individual minds tends to ignore the community-based experience of being forced into exile. Rupture occurs not only in the narrative thread running through each individual refugee's life, but also in their familiar social networks (Bracken, 1998: 38). With this break in community-based support and meaning-making, it is difficult to mourn individually what has been lost without reference to what has been lost at a social level. So, with few perceived alternatives, many individuals present medically with somatic expressions of their distress (ibid: 21). They are then given a diagnosis and treated individually without attention being paid to the fact that whole social structures have been destroyed around them. Not taking the lost social context into account may also be connected to an unconscious wish to keep control over the refugee in the new country.

My experience as the recipient of a great deal of socio-political trauma that could not be adequately explained or described, has taught me that what is experienced, but not acknowledged, becomes an internal nagging anger, vulnerability or loneliness, without words. Physical symptoms come and go but locating their origins in the transmitted trauma is difficult. They go on through life without end until the connections between the original political experience and the personal picking up of that often-undescribed experience can be made and described. The problem then is how to find a context to talk about what has become obvious to oneself but not to others, how to withstand a second level of silencing that resonates with the first, when one tries to point out the long-term results of this hidden oppression. It is in these situations that the larger group can be so helpful.

Patrick de Maré, the British group analyst who was concerned with revealing the dialectic between the individual and the social context, drew attention to the way prevailing cultures tend to prevent us from thinking certain thoughts (de Maré, Piper, & Thompson, 1991: 77). My own experience of growing up in a culture that could not help me find a way to describe my experience, left me without words. This state was further reinforced by a culture that applauded stoicism and denigrated victimhood, ensuring that the social trauma I carried remained hidden and almost impossible for me or anyone else to acknowledge. Assmann takes on this dilemma in her book and inquires into the way such events are remembered individually, how they are passed on or silenced as collective experience, how they are publicly recognised and in what forms of media and ritualised commemorations they are being continually reconstructed. Psychological attitudes, political constellations and cultural conditions of processes and remembering are particularly important as are normative frames of reference and the possibility (or impossibility) of making comparisons (Assmann, 2016: 4).

The larger group, with its focus on the social experience of individuals, is one such place where socio-political traumas such as mine can emerge and be witnessed in a social context, often for the first time. There, it is possible to observe emerging dominant and oppressive cultures that silence; it provides not only an opportunity to gain what de Maré refers to as 'outsight,' as opposed to insight into these experiences, but also the possibility of repair (de Maré, Piper, & Thompson, 1991: 129). It's where I feel most at home, where the diverse group reflects my diverse history and I return to it again and again.

Afterword

Since presenting this paper in Belgrade in 2018, my thinking has taken a deeper turn. There were clues in what my father told me that I was unable to take in fully. Metabolising transgenerational trauma takes a long time. It centres around my father's humiliation, not once by being forced to leave Germany, but twice by being brutally deported from the country he thought had given him refuge. He never used the word humiliation, he just puzzled about feeling shame. Although obvious that he had suffered humiliation in retrospect, it had never really crossed my mind until I came across the following definition recently. Humiliation is a demonstrative exercise of power against one or more persons, which consistently involves a number of elements: stripping of status; rejection or exclusion; unpredictability or arbitrariness; and a personal sense of injustice matched by the lack of any remedy for the injustice suffered. Such a definition makes it easier to identify when humiliation has taken place, to understand the feelings that result from humiliation and to distinguish humiliation from shame. Humiliation leads to a strong sense that one has been wronged, while shame involves a sense that one has done wrong and diminished oneself in one's own eyes or in the eyes of others. (Leask, 2013: 131).

Leask also quotes Hartling and Luchetta (1999: 263) who suggest, "shame can serve an appropriate adaptive function by inhibiting aggression or protecting an individual from unnecessary personal exposure." For the first time, I understood that the shame my father felt was a way of protecting himself from excruciating reminders of humiliation that he had sought to avoid his whole life. Making this connection allowed something profound to shift in me. As his beloved daughter, I no longer needed to take on his transmitted burden, but instead, I felt a rush of my own sadness for him.[1]

Note

1 A paper on a similar theme was published in the *Transactional Analysis Journal*, Vol. 49 (4), 233–247, 2019, Routledge, 'Socio-Political Trauma: Forgetting, Remembering and Group Analysis'.

References

Arendt, H., 'We refugees'. *Menorah Journal*, 31:1, pp. 69–77, 1943. http://www.documenta14.de/en/south/35_we_refugees.

Assmann, A., *Shadows of Trauma: Memory and the Politics of Postwar Identity* (trans. Clift, S.). New York: Fordham University, 2016.

Bracken, P., 'Hidden Agendas: Deconstructing Post Traumatic Stress Disorder', *Rethinking the Trauma of War*, Ed: Bracken, P. & Petty, C. London: Free Association, 1998.

Dalal, F, *Race, Colour and the Processes of Racialization: New Perspectives from Group Analysis, Psychoanalysis and Sociology*. Hove: Brunner-Routledge, 2002.

de Maré, P, Piper, R, Thompson, S, *Koinonia: From Hate, through Dialogue, to Culture in the Larger Group*, London: Routledge, 1991.

Glyn-Blanco, R., McLintock, M., & Papazymouri, D., *The System of Systems*. Athens: Self Published, 2017.

Hartling, L., & Luchetta, T., 'Humiliation: Assessing the impact of derision, degradation, and debasement'. *Journal of Primary Prevention*, 19, pp. 259–278, 1999.

Lafitte F., *The Internment of Aliens*. London: Penguin, 1940 & 1988.

Leask, P., 'Losing trust in the world: Humiliation and its consequences', *Psychodynamic Practice: Individuals, Groups and Organisations*, 19:2, pp. 129–142, 2013.

London, L., *Whitehall and the Jews, 1933–1948: British Immigration Policy, Jewish Refugees and the Holocaust*. Cambridge: Cambridge University Press, 2001.

Pedahzur, A., *Suicide Terrorism*. Cambridge: Polity, 2005.

Rampen, J., 'Britain's treatment of refugees fleeing the Nazis is a story of brutality cloaked in bureaucracy'. New Statesman, 2018. https://www.newstatesman.com/politics/uk/2018/01/britain-s-treatment-refugees-fleeing-nazis-story-brutality-cloaked-bureaucracy

Taylor, B., & Ferguson, K., Refugee history: The 1930s crisis and today. Protection Approaches, 2017. https://img1.wsimg.com/blobby/go/131c96cc-7e6f-4c06-ae37-6550dbd85dde/downloads/Refugee%20History%20the%201930s%20crisis%20and%20today.pdf?ver=1591696811585

Tisdall, S., 'Europe must make Trump pay for trashing the Iran deal'. The Guardian International Edition, 9 May 2018, pp. 1–2, 2018.

Wiesel, E., *Night* (trans. Wiesel, M.). New York: Hill and Wang, 2006.

Chapter 2

Recovering Dignity

The Remarkable History of Dr Rosenberg and Dr Goldowski

Wojtek Hanbowski

The Hospital in Obrzyce

This story begins in the eastern part of Germany in 1900 with the building of a modern mental hospital in Obrzyce, which is now a part of Poland. In an area of 114 hectares, a complex of modern and spacious house was developed. Initially, the Fourth Posen Regional Obrawalde Hospital for Mad People (4 *Posenschen Provinzialirrenanstalt Obrawalde bei Meseritz*) admitted 700 people, but within 10 years it had become a huge institution for 2,000 patients. There were admission wards, wards for quiet patients, for mildly quiet patients, for unquiet patients and for especially unquiet patients as well as a unit for untreatable patients. Gradually, other departments were opened: radiology, gynaecology, midwifery and detoxicology (Dramowicz 2004).

Although the hospital name "for Mad People" may suggest an inhumane attitude towards mentally ill people, the classification of patients from quiet through to untreatable was actually a means of properly allocating patients in the hospital system. It was not a way of prejudicially diagnosing patients but rather an attempt to ensure that patients were placed in a proper and appropriate therapeutic setting. The patient pavilions were spacious and comfortable and the hospital grounds contained a sports stadium, a shooting gallery, two swimming pools, an indoor sports arena and a cinema. Patients could work and learn under the supervisions of craftsmen in a bakery, in fabric workshops and on the huge hospital farm. The hospital had a modern system of telecommunication with underground phone and electric wires. There was a luxurious villa for the director and comfortable houses for doctors as well as a village for the nurses. The hospital was a self-contained system where staff were able to do their work in comfort and with support, and patients could develop their skills and live with dignity. When it was observed that children were sometimes abandoned by their mothers in the midwifery ward, an infant and children unit was opened. From its foundation until the beginning of the Second World War the hospital was run with the humanitarian aim of treating people with respect and offering them the best care.

DOI: 10.4324/9781003269649-4

In the 1930s, the German legal system allowed for the sterilization and, later, the extermination of people judged to be "life, unworthy of life"; in effect this was a programme of mass murder, including that of mentally ill people. Perversely this was called "euthanasia," a corruption of the Greek term for helping somebody who wished to die with dignity. Initially, this programme of mass killing was implemented in central Germany, but after public outrage and the intervention of the Catholic and Protestant churches, it was moved out of sight to Germany's eastern border.

Thus, mass killing came to Obrzyce. Between 1942 and 1944, more than 10,000 people were killed mainly with injections of a mixture of morphine and scopolamine (Dramowicz 2004). There were doctors who refused to participate in this programme and they were allowed to continue their work in other areas; nevertheless, we can only imagine how these dramatic changes radically effected the philosophy of the hospital, demoralized its staff, and what the patients felt as they waited for their execution in hospital.

The Events of 1945

The Nazis not only murdered their own citizens, they dehumanized Jews, Poles and eventually the Russians as *Untermenschen*, or "inferior people." The atrocities committed on an industrial scale are infamous. When the tide of war turned, the Russians were equally determined on the total destruction of the German nation and on the imposition of a political system that denied individuals and nations the dignity of self-determination. Their terrible treatment of the people they came across as they swept towards Berlin is also well documented (e.g. Moran 2008). In Obrzyce, 10,000 of the 12,000 German inhabitants of the town left before the Russians arrived out of fear of what would happen to them should they fell into Russian hands. Most of the staff of the hospital fled, leaving the patients to fend for themselves. It was at that point that a German dentist, Dr Rosenberg, a patient at the hospital, began to organise food distribution, cooking and heating rotations within the hospital and generally to ensure that the remaining patients, many of whom were physically and mentally incapacitated, were able to be fed and kept warm (this was in January). Like the other patients, he had been sent to Obrzyce to be exterminated; I have been unable to ascertain why.

What I am about to recount occurred in the context of the clash between two systems that were in a murderous conflict with each other. At that time and in that part of the world, prejudice was truly deadly. I am indebted to an account of what happened in the hospital after the arrival of the Russians to a document written by Dr Rosenberg, discovered in the 1990s by the Polish archivist Joachim Bohe.

When the Russians arrived at the end of January 1945, they were commanded by an Army colonel known to me at this point only as Dr Goldowski. His first actions upon taking command of the hospital was to segregate his own soldiers from the patients—largely it seems to protect the patients, particularly the female patients. He then began to investigate the situation he had inherited.

Dr Rosenberg describes his first meeting with Dr Goldowski:

> One evening, during supper time, the door opened and a number of Russian officers came in. They were headed by a strikingly handsome Staff officer wearing a tall Crimean cap. He asked in German „ Where is Dr Rosenberg?" When I introduced myself he took me outside, told me he was a doctor and asked me about the situation in the hospital. The next morning he ordered me to go to his quarters, he lived in Villa number 11, where we discussed the existing situation. He praised me for having, on my own initiative, organised the care of the ill patients and told me that he was appointing me officially as the Director of the Hospital.

Despite this promising beginning, enmity between the Russians and the Germans within the hospital was barely contained: a Russian soldier was killed by a sniper in the hospital grounds, two of Dr Rosenberg's appointed staff were captured by another Russian unit and were only just saved from transportation to Siberia and Russian soldiers regularly tried to break into the women's villas. Large parts of the hospital amenities had been converted into a hospital for wounded Russian soldiers and there was constant tension about scarce resources of food and heating being allocated to the German patients. Some of the German hospital staff who had fled were captured and were brought back to Obrzyce. This is Dr Rosenberg's account of what happened to three of them:

> A. Ratajczak (a female German nurse who had been heavily implicated in the killings at Obrzyce) was put before a Russian military court and together with the male nurse Guhlke, who was also found guilty, were on the basis of that judgement executed by firing squad. On the basis of varied evidence it was clear to the same court that the Medical Advisor to the hospital Dr Vollhaim had always been against the euthanasia programme and had never participated in it. His unshakeable belief in his principles in such difficult circumstances was recognised by the Russians.

I do not have space to tell you of all the struggles that Dr Rosenberg and Dr Goldowski endured to ensure that the Germans in the hospital were provided with adequate care. Despite constant hardship and in the terrible context of what had happened and was happening as the Russians advanced on Berlin, the patients in Obrzyce were able to live safely until the end of the war. In his account, Dr Rosenberg is clear that this was largely due to the humanitarian stance of Dr Goldowski to whom he dedicated his account with gratitude and respect.

Dr Goldowski

I wanted to learn more about Dr Goldowski. My psychoanalytical ethos, the inspiration of Joachim Bohe's work and that of the famous film *Searching for Sugar Man,* by Malik Bendjelloul, whose efforts rediscovered the forgotten singer Sixto Rodriguez, encouraged me to believe that research always has a sense and may uncover unexpected findings.

I started, as people do in these days, with Google and instantly found just one name for Goldowski with the correct initials: E. D. An address was given in the documentation I discovered: the military hospital in Kiev. I learnt from Igor Kadyrov, my psychoanalyst colleague based in Moscow, that the Russian military hospital in Kiev is a very old, large and well-known Institution, now in Ukraine. Another colleague, Dr Rostyslav Hryvul from Lvov, brought to me, by bus (!), five huge leather-bound volumes on the 250-year history of the hospital (Boytschack 2009). Seven of these large pages are devoted to Dr Evsiej Davidovitch Goldowski.

He was born in 1892 in Kiev. His father was a well-known painter and architect and Evsiej Davidovitch himself began to study art and medicine, but eventually he concentrated on medicine. His passion for painting never disappeared. He had six brothers and four of them became doctors, two engineers, and the last one an economist. He spent more than 20 years at the military hospital where he ran a neurology unit and where his personality and skill made him something of a legend. He was a highly educated and cultured man with a fantastic photographic memory. He spoke fluent English, French, German, Spanish and Polish. Sport was one of his passions. He liked rowing and is still considered as one of best-ever tennis players to have played on the hospital's courts.

In the 1920s and 1930s, Kiev's military hospital was a prestigious institution and hence Dr Goldowski gave the hospital address in the document we discovered. There, he treated patients, taught doctors, pursued his research and introduced many organizational and clinical innovations. He was a respected and active member of the doctor's organization. He was interested in the impact of military systems on the psychology, morale and ethos of officers and doctors. He insisted on a close cooperation between civil and military doctors as a means of humanizing the military approach. He tried to develop new forms of treatment for neurosis. Physical exercises were recommended and he introduced drawing books for the patients. The patients were asked to express their feelings and thoughts in drawings, which were then discussed and analysed.

During the Second World War Dr Goldowski held the post of a General Neuropathologist of the Soviet Army in Germany. Towards the end of the war, partly because of his knowledge of languages and his intelligence, he was stationed in Marshall Zukov's headquarters. He lived in Berlin until 1948. His second daughter was born there in 1945, the first one was born in 1942. He also had a son, who like his grandfather was an architect and like his father a painter. In 1948, Dr Goldowski was nominated as head of all military sanatoriums in Crimea and moved to the beautiful town of Eupatoria on the Black Sea coast. He died in 1952, at the age of 60, from a brain tumour, which he diagnosed himself. He was buried in the Jewish cemetery in Eupatoria but his grave has not survived.

In the history of Kiev's military hospital, I found a short and remarkable note. It stated that during the Stalinist purges of the Bolshevik Party, Dr Goldowski was expelled but then re-instated on appeal. It gave a reason for his sacking from the Party: it was his passionate interest and devotion to the ideas of Sigmund Freud!

The document we found in Google that gave the address of Dr Goldowski was the German version of the International Psychoanalytical Association Roster from 1927 to 1929 (Bulletin of the IPA 1929). Thus, I discovered that Colonel, Dr Evsiej Davidovitch Goldowski was a psychoanalyst, an associate member of the Russian Psychoanalytical Society.

The Russian Psychoanalytical Society

Although the short history of the Russian Psychoanalytical Society is well documented, the fact of its existence is not now widely remembered. Psychoanalysis became popular among Russian doctors with Freud's first publications. In 1912, Freud wrote to Swiss psychiatrist Carl Jung: "In Russia (Odessa) there seems to be a local epidemic of psychoanalysis" (Etkind 1994, p. 191). In 1922, the Russian Psycho-Analytical Society was established by the Ministry of Education (Etkind 1994, Kadyrov 2005). It was received enthusiastically by the international psychoanalytical community. It was the first society to receive state support. In 1923, the Society became a component of the International Psychoanalytical Association (IPA) and among its first leaders were Alexander Luria, Mosche Wulff, Ivan Ermakoff and Sabine Spielrein who all settled in Rostov in 1923 after returning from Geneva, Switzerland. The Society received support from Trotsky who had known Dr. Victor Adler in Vienna and who had a great respect for psychoanalysis. Between 1923 and 1930, the Russian psychoanalysts were very active. In Moscow, they ran a children's home and a psychoanalytical clinic, following the example of the Berlin Clinic for Psychoanalysis.

Above all, they organised scientific meetings. The topics are as contemporary now as they were then: for instance, the psychology of idealism, the psychoanalysis of artistic creation, hate and the death instinct. Spielrein spoke on child analysis. There were also lectures on the psychoanalysis of religion, on the development of the epistemophilic instinct in a child and papers on the application of the psychoanalytic method in literature. Other contributions examined whether psychoanalysis contradicted dialectic materialism, Sinology and psychoanalysis and the application of psychoanalysis to art.

These are just few of many titles from a very rich scientific programme and one can see a broad spectrum of interest. However, after Trotsky's denunciation as an enemy of the state and his emigration, the fortunes of the Society changed dramatically and finally, in the 1930s, the Society disappeared.

The 10 years of existence of the Russian Psychoanalytical Society shows a group of creative, passionate and very active people led by a conviction that the human mind can be explored and treated with respect. The records of the society show that Dr Goldowski was a frequent participant at scientific meetings. I do not know what personal analysis he underwent since, at that time, training systems were not in place. (I can only be sure that two members, Spielrein and Wulff, had their own analyses.)

Nevertheless, I end by suggesting that Dr Goldowski had a humanity that manifested itself in his psychoanalytic and scientific predisposition. This drew him to psychoanalysis in the first place, was further developed in his psychoanalytical society, and was fully demonstrated by his dignity, courage and conviction in Obrzyce in 1945.

Psychoanalysis

The reparative processes in therapy and in life run in difficult ways, or sometimes they cannot emerge, if the psychological life revolves around various forms of revenge fantasies.

Especially is the case when revenge by the harm suffered is identified with reparation. We then deal with a vicious cycle in which revenge is justified by harm, which in turn is "nurtured" because it justifies revenge and frees the individual from feeling guilty.

John Steiner (1996) locates the roots of pathological revenge in the Oedipal situation, in which the child, recognizing a close relationship between the parents, experiences it as rejection. The grudge established in this period may shape a predisposition to experience permanent harm and the desire for revenge. Steiner also points out that the sense of harm and the desire for revenge are factors that create an unusually strong bond with the object. In turn, the ability to forgive is always related to the possibility of experiencing separation. If we are able to separate ourselves from the object, then we are also able to tell ourselves: go your own way, everything has been evened out. Nurtured harm connects with the object forever, because rarely can revenge attain its fulfilment.

The history of individuals and groups is familiar with many examples of harm and losses, which gave rise to equally beautiful initiatives, restoring people's dignified relationships as well as starting a sequence of destruction.

The events described by me from the hospital in Obrzyce were a good example of how people can strive for cooperation and reconciliation by overcoming prejudices.

However, the history of individuals and groups is also familiar with many examples of how good reparative intentions and the search for justice can turn into a vengeful and destructive action. Steiner writes:

> I came to the conclusion that revenge is a complex phenomenon. It often appears to begin with a real or imagined wrong which provokes no more than a wish for justice and a reasonable compensation. The demand for revenge is particularly pressing when the injury and wrong has been done not only to the self but also to good internal objects which are represented by the family or group. The conscious aim of the revenge may then be to clear the good name of the injured object and to restore the family honour. Revenge here begins as an expression of the life instinct, and demands that we stand up against those who injure us and threaten our objects.
>
> In practice, justice is seldom able to intervene in an adequate way, and its failure to give satisfaction allows other motives to become attached to the initially just cause. Old hatreds, based on narcissistic wounds, greed, jealousy, Oedipal rivalries, and especially the primitive destructiveness rooted in envy, take over and give revenge its insatiable nature, with devastating consequences if it is not restrained. When the death instinct comes to dominate, revenge is not satisfied until the object and with it the self is totally destroyed.
>
> (1993)

A young female patient, an artist moving around the commercial sphere, came to psychoanalysis after her marriage due to numerous somatic conditions. She also suffered from a permanent feeling of unfulfillment and her creative ideas contained many motives of harm and revenge. She thought of herself as poorly educated, stupid and unattractive.

She had numerous siblings and blamed her parents for her failures, especially her mother, whom she described as intrusive. Whenever she was faced with any sort of failure or an event which she subjectively experienced as defeat, it instantly reminded her of her mother's behaviour, which she felt broke her character and now contributed to disasters.

The patient's suffering always indicted towards the mother's fault. This mechanism was transferred onto other relationships. Almost all disappointments were caused by pain and suffering for which the perpetrators of these disappointments were blamed. Once, shortly before a holiday break, the patient submitted her project to a well-known company. At first, she waited a long time for an answer, and then she learned that her project had arrived after the deadline and could not be considered.

Later, the company established contact with her and assured her that after the holiday period her project would be re-evaluated. Despite this, the patient came to the conclusion that the company was obviously misleading her, so she should withdraw her proposal herself. She therefore concluded that it makes no sense to submit the project again because it is proof of her lack of qualifications.

She also maintained that her analysis makes no sense because she is too stupid and doesn't know how to make use of it. During the sessions she was silent.

In the time of these deaf sessions, I felt helpless and had no ideas which would help to break the impasse. In the end, I tried to show the patient that submitting the proposal after the holidays was disappointing and humiliating for her. I suggested that she felt rejected by both the corporation and her analyst, who was soon starting a holiday break. I added that in this situation, the fact of admission after the holidays was not satisfactory for her and, in this way, she rejected herself: the analysis became meaningless and the company no longer interested her.

At the same time in Poland, there was a lot of tension around government proposals for changes in the legal system, which aroused a lot of controversy and resulted in demonstrations. I pointed out to the patient that she does not mention these events during the sessions. She said she did not understand the criticism of the government and did not want to join the protests despite them being located in areas near her. In several sentences she laid out her views, which largely sympathised with the philosophy of the governors. She spoke about social justice and the fact that it should be restored by depriving people of privileges obtained in an unjustified way. She expressed her sympathy for a politician who had lost his brother in a plane crash and criticism of those who hinder public commemoration of this catastrophe.

The patient clearly expressed her views, in which the feeling of hurt and vengeance prevailed and were directed toward those who either contributed to or used injustice. I commented on the convergence of her political and social views with the experience of herself and the people associated with her. This allowed us to understand the psychological system that had entangled the patient for years. In this system, the harm could only be repaired by revenge. In this philosophy, justice hinged on hurting the perpetrators. This, in turn, did not evoke guilt nor compassion for the victims of revenge as long as their own suffering lasted. By discussing these topics, the patient understood how her self-criticism and suffering, which deprived her of all life privileges, caused and were at the same time the result of jealousy and the desire for retaliation.

During the next sessions, neither I nor the patient referred directly to the previous ones. However, the patient became lively and talked a lot about many friends with whom she resumed contact. She also talked beautifully about nature, which she enjoyed in connection with her holiday plans. I commented on it as a feeling of regaining a good, beautiful and optimistic world that restores the purpose of effort and plans.

References

Boytschack, M.P., The History of Kiev's Military Hospital Kiev, 2009.
Bulletin of the International Psycho-Analytical Association, List of Members of the IPA. Russian Society, vol. 10, p. 561, 1929.
Dramowicz, Waldemar, Obrzyce. Dzieje Szpitala. Miedzyrzecz, 2004.
Etkind, Alexander M., How Psychoanalysis Was Received In Russia, 1906–1936. J. Anal. Psychol., 39: 191–202, 1994.
Kadyrov I.M., Analytical Space and Work in Russia: Some Remarks on Past and Present. Int. J. Psychoanal., 86: 1–16, 2005.
Moran, M., Country in the Moon. Granta Publications. London. 2008.
Steiner, J., Revenge, Resentment, Remorse and Reparation in Psychic Retreats. Routledge. London, p. 85. 1993.
Steiner, J., Revenge and Resentment in the 'Oedipus Situation'. Int. J. Psychoanal., 77: 433–443, 1996.

Chapter 3

A Wound Within a Wound Within a Wound

Social Dreaming in Jerusalem

OR Netanely, Hanni Biran, Judith Ezra, and Hanan Sabah Teicher

Social Dreaming

The social dreaming matrix is a group facilitation method formulated by Gordon Lawrence (2000). It is practiced in the psychoanalytic field as a professional workshop during conferences, or as an action-research method in organizational consultation. It is based on the assumption of a shared social unconscious that is manifested in the dreams of individuals in a given society or organization.

The Initiative

For the past six years, we've been conducting social dreaming matrices, inviting people from the local community in Tel Aviv to share their dreams with each other, in order to find a shared meaning to their unconscious thoughts. We held them in community centres and in art galleries, and published them in social media. Usually between 20 and 60 people attended, of all ages, and of various occupations. Recently, we held two matrices in the Jerusalem YMCA and felt it was a meaningful change.

In the matrices, we invited people to share their dreams and associations, as if each of them is holding an individual piece of a broader social puzzle—a social unconscious. After a bit more than an hour of dream-orgying," we took a break and then sat back down to discuss what personal experiences were taken from the matrix.

In this chapter, we will compare social dreaming from gatherings held in Tel Aviv to those held in Jerusalem.

Our Thesis

Analyzing the imagery of this hyper-echoing dream space, we arrived at some formalizations of the content that came up—of the social unconscious phantasy.

DOI: 10.4324/9781003269649-5

We claim that the dreams are an attempt to organize a social reality of a complex conflict that leads to an unknown future, which somehow tends to continue the conflict.

First, we saw that this complex reality is organized by an attachment to two symbolic categories: gender and generation. These two symbolic categories connect the individual level to a greater whole, the social level.

We then recognized a triangle form, with two vertices representing the conflict, and the third vertex representing some sort of resolution. For example, a conflict between two genders, resolved through the formation of a third—an offspring. We will discuss the variations on the third vertex. We named the variations: romantic, nostalgic, and emergent.

In the romantic version, the conflict resolution is invested in the next generation. The nostalgic resolution of the conflict is invested in a dead father figure. The emergent resolution depends on a perspective change to a higher level of consciousness.

We will discuss the interchangeable romantic and nostalgic third vertex, and argue that offspring and ghosts serve the same function—to provide a false sense of familiarity to unpredictable continuity. We will argue that this equation of offspring with ghosts, facilitates the sacrifice of the next generation.

Finally, we will discuss the emergent third vertex, as a superimposed teleology of development. We will argue that whether emergent processes are a form of development or degradation is unclear.

Tel Aviv Hopes for the Future

Tel Aviv is a liberal city, so much so that it is criticized for being an isolated bubble, detached from Israel's harsh socio-economic and political conflicts.

Matrix #1

There seemed to be a lot of dreams about uncanny otherness, and an effort to pin down who the Other is. Ethnic and political splits surfaced in the dreams. Two symbolic differences that held a lot of attachment value for the dreamers were generation and gender. Though people thought to be different in generations and genders competed with the opposing categories, like in the case of ethnic splits, they still reserved a connection to the opposing identity and cared for the greater whole, unlike in the case of ethnic splits. For example, the younger generation could blame the older generation for the mess they inherited from them, but parent-child connection would still be something very clear to hold on to in all the confusion. One of the matrices converges into this final dream:

> I dreamed that I am going to Egypt, and I am worried. I am afraid that the Egyptians will see that my face looks like my father's—and he

> fought in Egypt, in the Sinai War. But then I see that there are women and children there and that their faces all look like my father's. They can see that I look like him and, to my surprise—they respect me for the fact that my father fought for something he believed in.

In this dream, we can see how our escape from our history and our alienation to our neighbours are related to one another. Haunting guilt for the sins of the father, is deterring the dreamer from connecting with his "war-brothers." The dreamer expects his identity to be something sterile and clean, to be free from the past and from the conflict that was before him. He discovers instead, that there is more fertile potential in contact, even if through violent conflict.

Matrix #2

In the next matrix held in Tel Aviv, anxiety about natural catastrophes turns into romantic complementarity between male and female genders. The thematic tensions culminate in the idea of "survival marriage" that appear in a final dream:

> In my dream, me and my family are going to visit my grandfather, who is a holocaust survivor, and had already passed away. He lives on the top floor and I realize that it is heaven, the afterlife. My grandfather married my grandmother after losing a wife and a daughter in the holocaust. In my dream, he has a new wife. Living with my grandmother was hard for him, it was a "marriage of survival". In my dream, me and my father come and sit on the couch in grandpa's living-room and we go into his new wife's robe. I put my arm in the left sleeve and my father puts his arm in the right sleeve, and we slip into it together.

This dream has many layers of meaning folded into it. The Holocaust is the apocalypse in the background, and the grandfather first married the grandmother in order to survive. This idea itself is very powerful—that people became couples to survive after their families were murdered and their world was ruined in the Holocaust. It is similar to the tale of Noah's ark, where animals boarded the ark in couples in order to survive the flood. In the case of Noah and his sons, the peace after the flood is distorted by incest. In this dream, too, the grandfather was unhappy in his romantic solution that allowed him to survive. This totemic grandfather requires a lot of solace. A survival marriage, then a love marriage, but that is not enough, even in the afterlife; when he is supposed to be happy in heaven, he needs the comfort of his offspring to be complete. The dreamer and her father fold together into the robe of the new wife, the two generations unite as an incestual couple, only to serve as a wife for the dead grandfather, thus collapsing another level of separateness and taboo, preparing to unite with him. It is as if they were chromosomes rolling back together to un-divide, in reversal of time, and return to their origin.

As we can see, in these matrices, held in Tel Aviv, the romantic solution and the nostalgic solution are interchangeable. Hope lies in the next generation, but sometimes the previous generation retains authority over the future.

Jerusalem Lives with its Ghosts

The city of Jerusalem, is the core of a multifaceted conflict—religious, ethnic, social, spiritual, etc. A conservative status quo holds it tightly from erupting. If a match is struck there, the whole world could ignite, and if peace could be found there, peace would be possible.

Matrix #1

In the first matrix, it is clear that in Jerusalem, the next generation does not promise hope. Participants share dreams about getting a baby to keep, and forgetting about it, only to find it dead. Another dream of childbirth ends with the mother looking at the baby looking back at it, only to see that the baby is hollow—like a circular, Escher version, of a matryoshka doll.

Instead, the living turn to the previous generation and their ghosts for hope. The following dream attracts a series of similar dreams after it:

> I have a dream from almost forty years ago, the night after my father died, I dreamt that we were all sitting in the living room and crying, like it was when we heard he died … and then he comes in a white cloak, and he is very angry that we made him dead. I felt very guilty but then relieved that he was alive.

An abundance of dreams about the resurrected dead follow this dream. A brother fallen in the war. Some premonition dreams about brothers, mothers, and fathers that would later be followed by news of their deaths in reality. In one dream, a dying mother is rejuvenated and becomes passionate with life in the retirement home, while her young daughter is buried in work. A dreamer buys sweaters for her long-dead brother, and she is insulted that he rejects the gift. The sweaters are a size too small for him, since he continued to grow after his death. Another father returns in a vision and says to his daughter: "I can't tell you more, only that we return from death, for now we have to stay in this place beyond recovery." The body of another father, a Holocaust survivor, was brought from the US to be buried in Jerusalem, according to his lifelong wish. He comes back in a vision within the dream, to comfort his grieving daughter and tells her that the place, Jerusalem, will give her solace. Thus, wishing her to live where he wished only to be buried. The sequence ends with a dreamer who is the father of four soldier sons. He dreams he has to go back and join the army to rescue his sons from captivity.

This series of dreams carries a strong nostalgic tone (and a desperate undertone). Unlike the dreams we saw in Tel Aviv, where the father figures were mostly conflictual, here the resurrected totemic fathers are very missed—idealized. They are so potent and hold so much power over the living, that they can even comfort the living for their own passing. We see this attitude as a major difference between liberal (young) Tel Aviv, that puts its hope from the future, and traditional (old) Jerusalem, that draws its hope from the past.

This interchangeability of future and past is troublesome. The trouble starts when we say that in the unconscious phantasy, there's a similar role for our offspring and our ghosts. Instead of sacrifice being in the past, and allowing survival into the future, they mix. The past survives while the future is sacrificed.

Matrix #2

The question of emergence is intertwined with the question of what lives over the grave of what has died: our genes through our offspring, our souls or our ghosts, our memes, or our influences on the broader whole of society. This dream opened the matrix:

> Tonight I dreamed that I'm going to the zoo … and the animals were mixed together: a bear with a lion and a zebra, all in the same cage. I didn't understand how it could be possible. Then after a few minutes humans came out of the animals. They told me, or that I somehow knew associatively, that the body belongs to an animal … but they did some sort of a brain transplant … and the human went into the animal. They stole the animal's body, and put a human brain into it. I started to cry in the dream, and went into hysteria. Then I got to a dolphin reef, that I lived in. Until suddenly a crazy underground water current started spewing dinosaur bones at me, with other bones of ancient animals that didn't exist. Then I woke up with my heart heavy on me, and inside I was sad.

In this apocalyptic dream, the wolf shall live with the lamb, because they share human minds. It might have been optimistic to hope that our intelligence will raise us above our violent animal nature. Instead, the emergence of intelligence is violent, monstrous. The dreamer then switches to a harmonic setting: swimming with dolphins. Dolphins have evolved with brains as big as ours, and have very sophisticated social lives, but they don't make war machines like us. The comparison to dolphins undermines the hope that all we need is a smart solution. The barrage of ancient bones of extinct species undermines a teleological view of evolution as leading to progress, that ends with human superiority. It reminds us that evolution goes through extinction on the way to survival.

> Lately I've been having such cruel dreams that I decided to stop fearing them because I understand that I am a conduit for the dream. Tonight, before dawn, I dreamed that I was supposed to go down a steep slope in the road, with some sort of vehicle. In front of me some Vespa is driving. I have some people with me in the car. I see the Vespa going down the slope, and reach a pothole in the road that's full of water. The Vespa and its rider get swallowed in the pothole, and he somehow manages to get up and climb out of the pothole. And I am thinking how will I manage to get up and climb out, because I'm carrying too much weight with all the people in the car. Then I think I don't need all the people to go down with me, their heads are enough, their bodies—well, I don't know ... So I take out a large knife and I chop the heads of the people who were with me in the car. Then I awoke.

Decapitation can be viewed as isolating the driving force of a person—the head as an *élan vital* (life force). Removing it from the redundant physical-biological form, would allow it to emerge from its corporal constraints and incorporate as an abstract part of a social whole. While a single vespa (wasp) can emerge from the puddle single-handedly, in order for the hive-mind to emerge, the members of the collective need to drop dead weight—their bodies. It seems that the social dream matrix is only partially able to contain a social consciousness, and that being incorporated into such a broader entity entails anxiety of losing individuality itself, by being thus divided.

The hive-mind itself is headless a headless cannibalistic monster. For the individual, it is a chaotic, Dionysian experience, denying individual choice and meaning. Unlike the phantasy of purposeful emergence, we don't really know whether the ascent in level of scale or complexity will resolve the conflict or degrade the little sense we have left. We need the body to own our pain and to empathize with the pain of others, and when disembodied we may become senseless vessels—but of what?

Discussion

In her book, "The Third Reich of Dreams," Charlotte Beradt (1964) describes the rise of fascism through the dreams of Jews in 1930s Germany. She describes the dreams becoming less personal and more subordinate to a group psychology. Early in 1933, one Jewish dreamer has to give a Nazi salute, and his hand is raised with great effort. The Nazi officer in the dream dismisses the salute from a non-Aryan, and the dreamer is left stuck with a raised arm against his will. The pressure to objectify oneself, then to be rejected and to remain inhuman is at the heart of this dynamic. Much before direct violence is employed. The social level here is like a virus that uses the individual against his/her interests, expropriating the host's vital force to proliferate itself.

We fear that the fantasied constructs of romantization, nostalgization and emergence that provide hope in the conflicts and uncertainty we live in, may have a price. These narrative ploys of phantasy may act as gloss, as automatic Instagram filters. These ploys not only blind us from seeing complex reality for what it is, and lead us to an inhuman automation of group thought and false divisions, but also act as an aesthetic pleasure that begs to be realized. Like the cliche of romanticizing the heroism of dead young soldiers on populist newspapers, thereby calling for more.

We view our work, and the creation of a dream space for the community to meet in dialogue, as a different way to emerge from the individual to the social, and to find connections across meaningful divides. We view it as real hope of a higher level of interrelatedness that also respects its individual components. Hope is offered in this context, not from anywhere else, but from inter-being itself. Offering a dream to the matrix and seeing it get charged with significance by other people, or picking someone else's dream to represent my own emotions, requires a change of mindset. Relinquishing individual authorship and letting go of the possibility to grow through copyrights and reproduction, and instead entering an open source collaboration allows for meeting points with otherness to act as a true emergent third, a space for fertile dialogue.

References

Beradt, C., *The third reich of dreams*. Chicago: Quadrangle Books, 1968.

Biran, H., Ezra, J., Netanely, O., and Sabah-Teicher, H. "Are you sharing a dream?": Social dreaming in a community. In S. Long and J. Manley (Eds), *Social Dreaming – Philosophy, Research, Theory and Practice*, 131–143. London and New York: Routledge, 2019.

Lawrence, W.G., Social dreaming illuminating social change. *Organ. Soc. Dyn.*, 1(1): 78–93, 2000.

Chapter 4

Scenarios of the Social Traumata in the Post-Communist Romanian Cinema

Cristina Călărăşanu

Thinking about Trauma

As it may seem a cliche, I feel we have to look once more on the meaning of trauma. The psychoanalyst Caroline Garland (2007) asks herself in her book *Understanding Trauma: A psychoanalytical approach*, what is a trauma?

> Trauma is a kind of wound. When we call an event traumatic, we are borrowing the word from the Greek where it refers to a piercing of the skin, a breaking of the bodily envelope. In physical medicine is denotes damage to tissue. Freud (1920) used the word metaphorically to emphasise how the mind too can be pierced and wounded by events, giving graphic force to his description of the way in which the mind can be thought of as being enveloped by a kind of skin, or protective shield.

She adds that not all traumatic events are devastating, and the mind has a way of engaging in a variety of defensive strategies for protecting itself. What is happening in a trauma? A particular event breaks the filters and the mind is flooded with more than it can make sense or manage. There is a massive disruption in functioning, like a breakdown.

> Thus a trauma is an event which does precisely this: overwhelms existing defence against anxiety in a form which also provides confirmation of those deepest universal anxieties. My own view is that the ego, once traumatised, can longer afford to believe in signal anxiety in any situation resembling the life-threatening trauma: it behaves as if it were flooded with automatic anxiety.

We could say, approaching British psychoanalyst Wilfred Ruprecht Bion's terms, that when we deal with trauma, the alpha function has been broken and the mind is filled with chaotic, fragmented, unrecognisable sensations, called beta elements. Trauma, by definition, occurs when this work, this alpha functioning, is overwhelmed and unable to contain and digest.

DOI: 10.4324/9781003269649-6

One feature of the effects of the trauma is described by Garland:

> The process of containment links in particular with one very recognisable feature of the thinking of survivors, the flashback: the sudden gripping sensation that you are not just thinking about what happend in the past, you are actually reliving it in the present. I suggest that the flasback is the experience of the loss of the container: the internalised place, or vessel, or space, intimately connected with good early care, in which thinking-about-something can occur. (2007)

When we speak about trauma in the social-historical context of persecutory regimes, the psychoanalyst Jed Sekoff (2003) makes one very important point, that the power of this regimes emanates not only from their capacities for physical violence, but also through the disruption and distorsion of imaginative symbols generation:

> All totalizing powers demand control of the basic symbols of life—what clothes to be worn, what art to be displayed, what music shall be heard, what words and ideas may be spoken or thought. The banishment of space for imaginative living is the necessary vehicle for terror regimes to colonize social and psychical space.

Cinema and Psychoanalysis

After all, why cinema? And what does cinema have to do with psychoanalysis? One very interesting hypothesis is offered by Andrea Sabbadini (2003) in the introductive chapter to *The Couch and the Silver Screen*. He writes that in a more general sense, cinema and psychoanalysis share an area that we can refer to by the term *insight*, meaning 'inner-sight' or a kind of 'within-the-mind' seeing. A film, especially when it emphasizes a psychoanalytic understanding of unconscious dynamics, operates in this area of insight and offers a gradual release of awareness. Some concepts common to both cinema and psychoanalysis could be the screen memories, the projection, the free association (mostly visual in cinema and verbal in psychoanalysis) and dreams (as in 1931, Hollywood was described by Soviet writer, Ilya Ehrenburg as a 'dream factory'). Cinema has a privileged tie to our mental activities and emotional experiences, that:

> It is a type of mime of both mind and world … Breaking from the confines of photography and theatre, it is unique in its representation of an abundant world in motion …. there is a persistent sense that cinema imitates the movement of the mind, that there is a correspondence (however elusive) to be discovered between psyche and cinema.
>
> (Lebeau, 2001)

When I had first the idea of approaching the Romanian cinema post 1989, I gave the topic a lot of thought. One colleague from London had the idea of putting me in touch with a friend of his, curator and filmmaker, and fan of the Romanian cinema, Adam Roberts[1]. So, an exchange emerged between Adam, born in Bogota, Colombia and living and working for many years in London, and I, born in the communist years and living since then in Bucharest, Romania. We started by asking ourselves what we should expect from such an unusual dialogue. Finally, we both set as 'counterdreamers' (a term by psychoanalyst Donald Meltzer for psychoanalytic reverie that arises from the countertransference during the session in response to the analysand's own dream and phantasies) watching two films as we were in a free associative analytic session. The two films were *4 Months, 3 Weeks, 2 Days* and *The Death of Mr. Lazarescu.*

* * * *

4 Months, 3 Weeks, 2 Days, directed by Cristian Mungiu (2007), brings into sharp focus one of the most difficult interdictions of the communist regime, the abortion. Set in 1987, the plot of this film is simple: a young woman must procure an illegal abortion. The film starts with the pregnant girl (Gabita) and her roommate (Otilia), both students, preparing for a very significant transaction, one that carries enormous risk and danger. This is a place where abortion is illegal, and the penalties severe. As events slip further from control, the film subtly incorporates elements of a thriller without relinquishing its enveloping realism: a knife slipped into a pocket, a ringing phone unanswered, a man seemingly trailing through the night-time streets. Bucharest is an underlit labyrinth where every turn mirrors a choice that must be made, but the city itself suggests a network of hallways and each location powerfully contributes to a sense of alienation. Although the civil authorities play no role in the narrative, the hallway outside the hotel room in which the abortion takes place is a sinister realm filled with blood-red club chairs that seem to await the arrival of unseen officials.

CRISTINA CĂLĂRĂŞANU: I was thinking about relationships. Every human exchange is mediated by a bribery (money, cigarettes, etc.). The way to obtain any kind of service is to bribe. This way to relate is presented as a most usual and common way of living, beyond any doubts or questions. Even the abortion is the subject of a bargaining. *In that time, life seems more of a transaction, than an interaction.*

ADAM ROBERTS: Yes indeed, the director chooses to present an immersive picture of subsistence living, where all contact and interaction is about transaction, about the exchange of goods and favours. To lose concentration in this most serious game can come at very great cost. Clever and astute players stay in the game, losers simply disappear. This far removed from capitalism, in this place this is how the most meagre essentials are obtained. We learn the price of everything, that everything has a price. That is the context. Barter is an exchange, in which very slim advantage is always to be worked towards. From the perspective of a world of excess, this is not easy to comprehend.

CC: You talk about the black market and about barter as a game which people played better or worse. I see it as a survival skill, which can be very dangerous, if you are not good at it, you can be caught. There is a complementary contrast between The Outside and the Inside. The terrible grey landscape inviting to a violent melancholia (cold, trash, dogs barking, poverty, the queues from the grocery, etc.). There is a constant feeling of danger in the air, like an invisible enemy waiting in the dark—this feeling of being watched was not just a paranoia in communism, it was a reality of the controlling system. The Inside—small, dirty, suffocating spaces inviting a feeling of being trapped. The constant smoking, an only way to defy the interdiction and the oppression, makes even the sensation suffocating. Rooms are decorated in a hideous, crowded way indicating the importance of *things*. Having *things* (meat, cigarettes, alcohol) means having a bizarre sense of living.

AR: Regarding your point about inside and outside: there are for me also a womb-like associations in which inside stands in contrast to outside. You represent negative connotations for both, but ironically there might be some small positives in the sense of inside representing the possibility of containment/holding/interiority … and smoking can be seen as visible breath, as a tangible sharing of air, that connects us and joins us. But then, the constant anxiety, the nagging fear that no matter how carefully one might plan or anticipate the endless pitfalls and dangers, the risk of discovery and exposure to harsh elements is absolutely constant. Existential fear, like a gun held to the temple in a constantly deferred execution, is inescapable. Knowing the system, playing the system, being on top of the system means beating the other or being beaten by the other. Danger is ever-present. Every position and every statement are contested. In this place, paranoia is not abnormal, it is a form of sanity. The opposite of being held!

CC: Talking about the constant anxiety, I believe that the profound silence marks many significant symbols: the sexual abuse, the terror of being caught, the broken naivety, the killing, the unbearable feeling of guilt and fear, the darkness of memory. Even the final scene trades a pact of silence covering the abuse and the transgression of interdiction: *We won't talk about that ever again.*

AR: Talking about silence, in cinema I am often struck by how sound is used to displace awareness of the moment, and how silence can serve to underline it. It is as if only when background noise is removed or silenced that there can be thought. Or something like that. In this film, I am struck by the use of running taps and of flushing toilets not only as a way of avoiding surveillance, but also as a source of white noise, so unstructured and calming, a version of silence. It is about the difference maybe between listening and hearing, one passive and allowing regress to a better psychological place and the other active and controlling attention.

CC: I guess, this is not about a fight between good and evil, this is a way of living. There are not just good people and bad people in this story, it is a very mixed and complex picture.

AR: Yet the film does not blandly offer the simple contrast of a helpless innocent at the mercy of the system. The pregnant woman is far from honest, misleading even her helpful friend. The closest to honesty anyone gets is when they are silent. Gabita lies about how far the pregnancy has progressed, even when that is an objective fact that cannot be denied. She even lies about arrangements made for the room booking, as if she will not be found out! Otilia may be from a humble background, but she is cunning and may survive this life. Her boyfriend, whose demands for kisses and unprotected sex, even at the risk of pregnancy, reveals scant regard for her feelings. Indeed, the coldness of their exchanges sound more like barter than sweet nothings. And Mr. Bebe the abortionist (is this the same sick joke in Romanian I wonder?) is confident, shrewd and evidently experienced. He has the sullen focus of the long-term prisoner, of the seasoned poker player, of a torturer taking his time. The abortionist sizes these two young women up, and then makes his play. This is a pregnancy of four months. Abortion is illegal, more so at four months. Therefore, he demands sex with both women before the procedure. The women have no choice but to comply.

CC: Yes, the so-called good doctor, Mr. Bebe (Mr. Baby), is there to help, but no help comes without a huge price. In an oppressive society with iron walls where people are trapped, perversion serves at best any purpose. When you are not free, you must submit. When you are bargaining illicit things, you must pay the price. There is no choice, there are only facts. In not only the human nature or structure, is the system penetrating from outside a private individual's internal world and building perverted links.

AR: What strikes me most is that in *4 Weeks* there is very little of what we could call 'maternal' in any sense! There is no holding by anyone/thing, not for the foetus, nor for anyone. The only mothering in sight (at the dinner) is neutralized and marginalized at every turn. That may be the greatest source of the horror for me. I feel I could survive anything as long as I am in contact with the maternal. Otilia's pragmatism may be as good as it gets in that era and that place.

CC: We see in the grotesque scene of the mother's anniversary something that was very common in that era: small talk around the most insignificant subjects and great importance to conversations about food. The orality is the only way of connecting and a diffuse expression of affection. The mother tells us how she was very upset about the fact that she was buying (with great difficulty) salami for her son, yet he refused to eat it.

AR: Right! And they do not notice the mute, stunned silence of Otilia. The boyfriend is irritated, as he no doubts hopes only for unprotected sex and senses he may be denied it. Otilia needs comfort, but he may be the last person on earth to offer it.

CC: And the loving mother who intrudes to bring more food, the dessert. I feel that there is an implosion of feelings. No one talks about it. I believe that's actually a defence mechanism, an operative thinking, and the mystery and the suspense are part of the silent trauma construction going to an abrupt ending. The only statement is actually a question: *Have you buried him?*

AR: Horror of horrors: Mr. Bebe's instructions for the disposal of the foetus are precise: do not flush it down the toilet; instead go to a remote housing estate, go to at least the 10th floor and use the garbage shoot. Only then can they be sure to avoid detection. There is no ceremony for the disposal of this corpse. Only anxiety, and the perpetual fear of discovery and of scrutiny and punishment keep this lifeless bundle of matter company as it tumbles down into the silence. Impossible to imagine how such a situation could come to pass. That human life can survive in such a context is astonishing. No one seems exempt from the burden of apprehension, the complete denial of warmth. Temperatures seem stuck at absolute zero. By the time she has packed the dead foetus into her bag and travelled to the distant housing blocks and sought out an underused and bleak staircase, headed for the rubbish disposal chute, she is in all but total darkness. The light has leached from the world, the moral turpitude of the situation matched by the penumbral dark.

* * * *

The Death of Mr. Lazarescu, directed by Cristi Puiu (2005), tells the story of a widower, a man who lives alone, and who calls the ambulance complaining about his physical condition and must be moved from one hospital to another in order to obtain a diagnosis and relief from his condition. The movie is deeply grounded in the country's present-day reality and in a disenchantment with the failed promises of a post-Ceaușescu Romania. Nevertheless, the film transcends these concerns and addresses more existential questions in a surprisingly funny manner. The film begins as the portentously named Dante Remus Lazarescu, a retired professor, wakes up in the evening amidst the chaos of his apartment, to lovingly feed his many cats. Lazarescu wakes with a headache and calls an ambulance as he is concerned about a recent ulcer surgery. While waiting for the ambulance to arrive, he meets his neighbours, who are willing to help him up to a certain point but refuse to accompany him to the hospital. The rest of the film comprises Lazarescu's nightmarish journey through the night in Bucharest, moving from hospital to hospital, with a weary ambulance nurse, acting as his Virgil.

AR: Mr. Lazarescu is not well. He has sores on his legs, complains of head pain, abdominal discomfort, and his stools are runny. There is a lot wrong with him, maybe everything is wrong. All the same, he is not much given to complaining and allows himself to be shunted from hospital to hospital, without grumbling. In his situation, I'd make such fuss! He dresses and undresses on request, suffers the humiliation of loss of bodily control, and eventually a head shaving and clean up by women whose manner reminds me more of mortuary attendants than of pre-op nurses. Lazarescu becomes, over this one night, a body not a person.

CC: Indeed, the entire story is a continuous look at the cause and origin of the somatic suffering. We hear one after the other about the bowel, the liver and finally the head. Alcoholism, cancer, ulcer, neoplasm, hematoma, etc. A medical story that never touches at any point the personal history. The multiple diagnosis is a metaphor of alienation. Who is this man? The several ill parts of this body are his only curriculum vitae. The perforated ulcer is actually a metaphor for the perforated mind. Something very bad and toxic makes Mr. Lazarescu feel ill. Is not only the deterioration of his body, is the loneliness and the meaningless of his life. A man utterly depressed, he's complaining about the physical pain, misplacing the psychic pain on the somatic area of the body. *I have a headache* keep Mr. Lazarescu repeatedly says, and finally and the answer is one of irony: *it's good, that's means you have one.*

AR: He is indeed a problem in one way, a sick body, whose imperfections are no doubt severe. But he is also an opportunity for an increasingly bizarre and cruel set of hair-splitting bureaucratic objections. A system needs bodies with which to show itself. At one point he is all but unconscious, and yet unless he can sign a consent form then a life-saving (we presume) operation cannot proceed. The doctor will in no way budge from this Kafkaesque demand. Indeed, watching this film, Kafka is always in mind. The fate of Lazarescu is to be powerfully reminded of K trapped in the coils of *The Castle*. In what seems more or less like real time, followed every step of the way by the busy camera, Lazarescu falls foul of regulations that cannot be known, systems that change without notice, of officials whose only purpose is to obstruct and prevent.

CC: Yes, I'm thinking about Ferenczi's confusion of tongues. We are struck by the coldness of the medical staff, and sometimes even their loathing and hatred of their patient. Grandiosity and superiority seem more important than empathy. The system is more important than one man. The permanent insertion of one collective accident tragedy (happening in the same night) means that there's always a social superior purpose above the trivial singular destiny. The scientific, ideological language is empty of any kind of meaningful content and the absurd procedures you have endured, they are the substitute for real dialogue and are marks of absurdity. We must follow the rules by any means. Nobody really cares, papers are more important than humans. Showing empathy is equal to insolence and insubordination.

AR: It is striking that neither Mr. Lazarescu and his neighbours, nor even the doctors, nurses, paramedics, radiographers and surgeons are ever in any way in agreement about what exactly it is that ails Mr. Lazarescu! His condition is rather an opportunity to assert position in a complex pecking order. Is it gender, race or ethnicity at stake here? Or education or professional affiliation? What solidarity or complicity is on show? Perhaps none of these, for this is a comedy of manners, a comedy about people behaving badly, in a specific social context—or mostly so.

As I see it, the story is one about human degradation, the objectivation of a human being, treated as if it is just a set of cold and useless procedures. One moment of insight from Mr. Lazarescu is when, in answering the question: *Are you still nauseous?* he says: *No, I feel some kind of melancholia. I don't know why.* That is the last moment of lucidity, before the final loss of conscience and identity.

AR: Can we touch on the comedic aspects of this film? The surgeon who may save Lazarescu's life is called Anghel. Lazarescu's name invokes the biblical character who is famous for being dead, and even his first name is Dante, and he leads us down into the circles of hell ...

CC: Mr. Lazarescu has a very unusual combination of names, Remus (the myth of Romulus and Remus) and Dante (Inferno), symbols of the beginning and the end, a paradox. Is he dead or alive?

AR: The best joke then is that Mr. Lazarescu is inconveniently alive, but the system has a solution to that! This mordent comedic note conceals a satirical intent. Lazarescu may be alive the film seems to say, but will soon be dead, if only the paperwork can be sorted out. Bodies are just so much weight, a challenge and bother for servants of a system determined to offer nothing. In any case, no one knows anything about how to help Lazarescu, or if they do, they aren't letting on. The idea that there might be any deep-seated compassion among the clinical classes seems all but impossible ...

CC: Beyond Mr. Lazarescu's story, this is a precise X-ray of the Romanian society in the post- communist years, a society with very troubled identity, split between new and old, alienated and forced to decline her old roots, with no links and living a life nowhere. A reborn society dying of an invisible illness. The filiation is violently broked: *it's very hard to raise a child,* says Mr. Lazarescu, *my daughter is married and lives in Canada, Toronto* (that is so far, keeping in touch is impossible). There's a double time in the movie, *now and then*. The time is marked by only one night, but the slowness makes it fell like forever, out of time and space. Two historical times are visible co-existing through dissociation: now (cell phones, haircuts, verbal expressions, attitude, party etc.)—a modern, post-communist time; and then, with features of communism—the way the apartment is decorated, the cold inside, the poor food, the lights keep turning off, the clothes and the secret discussion about everyday issues (like buying alcohol). Fourteen years ago, he had an ulcer surgery and the traces of his pain are located in the past. *My headache comes from ulcer* Mr. Lazarescu keeps repeating. The past follows Mr. Lazarescu (old newspapers he never throws away).

AR: But is there perhaps one glimmer of light? Comedy surely demands as much. The paramedic, a woman, who faithfully, doggedly transports Lazarescu from hospital to hospital, who makes sure that the few diagnostic notes and scans are seen by doctors, who argues for urgency despite put-downs and humiliation at the hands of clerks, nurses and medics. She is someone who seems to offer some hope, even if at one point she tots up the likely cost of what Lazarescu has received. But on a final note, the cinematography is a triumph. The sickly greens, the miasmic, guttering flickers of light all but extinguished, even the jaundiced flicker of sodium light or of the fluorescent tubes of the clinical spaces evoke for the viewer a bodily sense of sickness and despair. It is impossible to remember as one watches that there might be the sunshine of spring or the dappled light of summer under shade. Here this is a perpetual night of the living dead.

* * * *

To conclude, or maybe to raise more questions about the ways of expressing trauma in the post-communist cinema, through the discussion with Adam—our interconnected and intercultural ideas and feelings—we've had a sort of discovery. One very interesting idea that strongly engaged my mind was Adam's association while watching the first film with the Julia Kristeva's (1982) concept of "abjection," described in *Powers of Horror*.

> The corpse, seen without God and outside of science, is the utmost of abjection. It is death infecting life. Abject. It is something rejected from which one does not part, from which someone does not protect oneself as from an object. [...] It is thus not lack of cleanliness or health that causes abjection but what disturbs identity, system, order. What does not respect borders, positions, rules. The in-between, the ambiguous, the composite. Abjection is immoral, sinister, scheming, and shady: a

> terror that dissembles, a hatred that smiles, a passion that uses the body for barter instead of inflaming it, a debtor who sells you up, a friend who stab you.

Another idea discussed with Adam, which could be as easy a consequence of the mechanism mentioned above, is the lack of any maternal sense or mothering linked with Andre Green's concept of the *dead mother*. We've thought that one of the effects is what we could name *'death mothering'*—a lack of any maternal feeling, result from an abusive and forced motherhood through the interdiction of abortion, but also through perverted links. People are bodies, not humans; the connection between the mind and the body being violently interrupted. There is emptiness, humiliation, sadism, dark melancholia, a lot of suffering, regression and orality is the only form of affection and social interaction. Having food is a sort of weird richness and giving food is the ultimate proof of love.

The confusion of tongues is the reference of a bizarre and cruel bureaucratic world, an absurd system where there are no subjects, only procedures and objects. After all, as Garland said, a trauma is a wound and for her to heal, we need a safe container. The ideological system is the lethal instrument of permanently attacking and destroying any king of containment.

Last, but not least, I would like to thank Adam for his warm reception of my invitation to watch the films and to share his lively thoughts with me. His voice has had the role of a third in a dyadic relation, which could have been easily corrupted by my own memories and feelings from the past.

References

Garland, Caroline, Understanding Trauma, A Psychoanalytic Approach, Karnac, London, 2007.

Kristeva, Julia, Powers of Herror: An Essay on Abjection, Columbia University Press, New York, 1982.

Lebeau, V, Psychoanalysis and Cinema: The play of shadows, page. 3, Wallflower Publisher, New York, 2001.

Sabbadini, Andrea, The Couch and the Silver Screen, Introduction, Routledge, London, 2003.

Sekoff, Jed, Witness and persecution in two short films, p. 79 of chapter 4 of The Couch and The Silver Screen, edited by Andrea Sabatini, Routledge, London, 2003.

The Death of Mr. Lazarescu, director Cristi Puiu, 2005.

4 Months, 3 Weeks, 2 Days, director Cristian Mungiu, 2007.

Part II

Group Identity and Social Trauma

Chapter 5

Group-analytic Identity Challenged by Social Trauma

Jelica Satarić and Bojana Mitrović

In this chapter, we shall discuss our experience: everything that has happened in Serbia and on the territory of former Yugoslavia over the last 30 years. It was a period of trauma and simultaneously the period when our group-analytic identity was formed. In 1991, we had mass demonstrations in Belgrade against then president Slobodan Milošević, Slobodan Milosevic was the president of Serbia while Serbia was one of the Yugoslav republics and during the wars in former Yugoslavia, from 1989 to 1997. He was also president of the Federal Republic of Yugoslavia from 1997 to 2000. He died in 2006, in Hague prison cell, before the trial in Hague tribunal was finished, with tanks on the streets, before the war even begun; 1991–1995 saw the breakup of Yugoslavia, wars in Slovenia, Croatia and Bosnia (Macedonia left the federation peacefully); in 1996 and 1997, months of daily protest rallies against Milošević occurred all over Serbia, conducing to economic and cultural isolation; in 1999, we saw the NATO bombing of Serbia and Montenegro and war in the Serbian province of Kosovo; in 2000, protests escalated to bring about the fall of Milošević; in 2003, the Serbian prime minister Zoran Đinđić was assassinated; in 2006, Montenegro declared independence and from that moment we are Serbia; in 2008, the Serbian province of Kosovo declared independence from Serbia. Today, Serbian borders are still not finalized and clear and we have been living in an economic crisis for decades. Many feel as if all this will never end, and as if we didn't have the time or strength to even clear out the debris.

Our discussions during the creation of this chapter are our specific experiences, which might be deeply connected to the topic itself. Reminiscing on our own experiences of the people from our personal, professional and social surroundings, as well as the information we had at our disposal, we once again relived the well-known feelings of injustice, helplessness, guilt, shame, grief and horror. We then fell into some sort of void of anxiety and fatigue, we were on the verge of giving up. Life seemed to drain from our thoughts, experiences and feelings, as if we stepped into our inner Pompei, into the space of strong emotions, which, in full swing of life, suddenly turned to stone. It was as if we didn't know how to share things we would

DOI: 10.4324/9781003269649-8

like to share, nor knew what we actually needed to share. One of the possible reasons for these strange oscillations is the fact that our group-analytic identity was developing in times of isolation and even though, over the last couple of years, we shared it with people from different surroundings, it is still difficult to get used to the fact that this kind of conference of the European Federation of Psychoanalytical Psychotherapists can be held in Belgrade today. At the time, we were developing as group analysts, such a thing was completely unimaginable, and it was hard to believe that it would ever really happen.

One of us had a dream that reflects numerous aspects of what we are talking about:

> "I'm in some large space that looks like a public space, but also an old flat. It's morning and it's still empty. I'm talking to Malcolm Pines about the EFPP conference in Belgrade. Then my phone starts to ring and I feel uncomfortable because Malcolm is alone while I'm on the phone. After that I'm talking to Haim Weinberg and I say to him: 'I think that I most of all carry the fear of whether everything will be all right.' I mean all right at the conference. Haim says that he thinks it's going to be a good and interesting event. We are together with two more colleagues and we are standing on the lawn, even though we are still inside the building. It's raining outside, Haim is leaving and going towards the crossroad in front of the building.
>
> I'm wondering if I have something to protect myself from the rain.
>
> Then I realize that we are in one of the two Yugoslav People's Army Headquarter buildings which were bombed in the NATO bombing in 1999.
>
> The building from my dream is partly ruined by NATO bombs, the other part is in use and it is the Serbian Ministry of Defense (the ruins of those two buildings are still at that crossroad, together with the buildings of the Serbian Ministry of Foreign Affairs and the Serbian Government)."

Malcolm Pines (1925–2021), was a group analyst and a psychoanalyst, a founder member of the Institute of Group Analysis and an honorary member of Group Analytic Society International. Dr Haim Weinberg, Ph.D, psychologist and group analyst. In time of great social traumas, group-analytic identity was very precious to us. We would not be exaggerating if we said that it played an important role in keeping our faith in people, in ourselves and others. (In the dream, us, group analysts, are standing in a place torn down by bombs, but we are alive, we are talking to our colleagues, we care for our professional community and we feel their support.)

Group-analytic identity as a professional identity is an aspect of our personal identity. However, group-analytic identity is also an aspect of our social identity, as the accepted group-analytic concepts, knowledge and practice refer to the primary social nature of man, sociality in general, to the group and collective processes and phenomena in which we find ourselves in various roles. In a social context, it is closest to the civil-democratic identity, sharing with it the democratic standards – pluralism, equality, freedom, respecting others and different others. It could be said that our social group-analytic identity is at the same time our civil-democratic identity, even though the other way around this can't be said. To wit, group-analytic identity surpasses the civil-democratic one with its further-reaching principles and expert knowledge.

Speaking about the conductor, S. H. Foulkes not only described the professional conditions to become a group analyst, but also the aspect of a group analyst's social identity:

> "… I would give a very high priority to the trainee's (future group analyst's) ethical integrity … honesty towards oneself and others is fundamental. There must be a love of truth, even if it is disagreeable and contrary to personal advantage … I do not mean that he should be a gregarious socialite, but a man open to new experiences and who is able to learn from them and to give himself a chance to experience his own responses to very different situations … He will have no undue expectations of having to be perfect (and, we would add, this is also not expected of others) and he will share the humility and modesty which as human people we have every reason to have … Whatever his own tastes and political convictions as a citizen, he must be liberal enough in a deep sense to treat all human people (in his group) as equal. This does not mean that they are not very different on a realistic level. (Some are attractive and charming, understanding; others difficult and annoying; some are influential and rich and others miserable creatures and even ugly). He need not blind himself to this, but in a profound sense we are equal human people …."
>
> (Foulkes, 1975)

Authentic feeling of equality of the different is one of the primary foundations of the group-analytic identity. It stems from the depth of the ethical aspect of human social nature. Equality is inseparable from freedom and responsibility. Acceptance of responsibility does not jeopardize equality. On the contrary! Dignity of a man who makes mistakes and tries not to repeat the same mistakes again allows him to change and mature. The same can be said for groups and societies. The group-analytic ideas of matrix and general connectedness do not lead to negating responsibility of individual groups and societies in the name of general responsibility. On the contrary, it accepts the responsibility of all groups and societies knowing that an individual, either society assuming or not assuming this responsibility, has consequences the entire community must bear. Equality of the different does not mean that the differences in power are not recognized, but in some way, it does mean that the more powerful ones must resign from their dominance, keeping in mind the dialectic nature of group dynamics. Is this pure idealization? Is it realistic to expect something like this in a social environment, both in the narrow and broader sense? Is an anti-group as equally rooted in human nature as a group, or is it just a consequence of an individual slowly becoming aware of the unavoidable connectedness and impossibility of permanent splitting on any grounds? We believe it is deeply rooted in human nature. According to group analyst Morris Nitsun, a group, as well as society, is not a static, defined essence; it lives in permanent play of various shapes and experiences. An anti-group is therefore created as a developmental phenomenon, i.e., a natural form of resistance against the group that has only one side, and points at its development in waves, oscillating between anti-group and pro-group. The pathological manifestation of anti-group can be found when the dialectical movement between these two forms of experience caves in, and the group gets stuck in one of them (Nitsun, 1996). Negative processes are an essential part of the society, but we must constantly search for the ways to accept responsibilities of both an individual and the society for something that has been done.

The period we are talking about is also the time of the collapse of the Federative state of Yugoslavia, which propagated precisely this fundamental value of group-analytic identity, the idea of equality of all peoples and nationalities. The time of our acceptance of our group-analytic identity is precisely this painful moment of facing not only the fact that this type of system could not survive, but that it also collapsed in bloody confrontations. Not accepting the reality and group dynamics, especially on the levels of power, opens up space for the creation of an anti-group. According to Nitsun, an anti-group represents the negative side of the positive processes within a group, which stems from basic fear and lack of trust in groups, and is expressed through various antagonistic processes within the group. In some cases, this cannot be solved in the usual way within a group, and it leads to its undermining and disintegration. In anti-group culture, the phenomenon of belonging to the group, the phenomenon of affiliation, can appear in two opposite forms—loss of affiliation on one side, or general and complete belonging on the other. Here, Nitsun refers to extreme religious or political groups in which there is an overwhelming identification with the ideology, the leader, and the group as an absolute society. There is no room for individuality. Instead of separating oneself from the others, there is a complete merging. This is related to the aforementioned topic of extreme cohesion. As it has been shown many times over, these groups end in self destruction. We can draw a conclusion that they hide separate anti-group attitudes which, the less visible they are and further away from the surface, become more and more devious. But there is a strong attraction in fundamentalism both in the East and in the West—to give one's identity over or to submit it to the almighty leader and the idealized totalitarian community or state (Nitsun, 1996). Maybe we could ask ourselves if we embraced the group-analytic identity in this fashion because that was the way to preserve at least a part of the values that were quickly vanishing before our eyes. Did we imbue it with ideals with which we were living and which were suddenly broken by trauma, not having been given enough time to enrich the reality of equality and get to know it better? This could be one of the challenges to our group-analytic identity. An anti-group can lead to a group falling apart, but the culture of said group can be preserved in the minds of its members. However, if an anti-group also leads to deep social trauma, in what measure can an individual be preserved from idealization on one hand, and de-idealization and apathy (anomy on a social level) on the other? Both of these, further down the road, leave room for the anti-group to strengthen. We remember the situations from several years ago when in our Group Analytic Society Belgrade there were misunderstandings and conflicts and some disillusioned members left the society. Many of us were also disappointed by those relations. We wonder how much de-idealization of us as group analysts and our society was there in this feeling of disappointment? Were we subconsciously expecting some form of "brotherhood and equality" from our former country? And where is the line between idealization and preservation of the very group-analytic identity? In this world full of various types of trauma, can it be said of us, group analysts, that we naturally seek out a place of "true equality"?

When Yugoslavia was falling apart, from our Yugoslav identity we felt ashamed and betrayed by all Yugoslav politicians and social groups and movements that we now feel were the carriers of the principles of anti-group, and who were promoting hatred and division of the country. We could not imagine just how much our (mutual) hatred would manage to destroy, embarrass and deeply divide us, Yugoslav people. However, some of us may have had an inkling of what was to come, as the Balkans are often referred to as "A powder keg." In the beginning of the World War II, Nikola Tesla said to Serbs and Croats: "Your hatred, transformed into electric power, could light many, many cities ..." Is it possible that the Yugoslav community founded on "brotherhood and equality of south Slavic peoples" was nothing but a lie, a forced, artificial creation? Deep down we cannot believe this. We remember Yugoslavia as it was right after the war.

Yugoslavia was not behind the iron curtain of the Soviet block and it certainly was not a Western democracy. It was not isolated although many of its citizens were isolated, persecuted or imprisoned for political reasons.

It was far from perfect but had many good sides, especially when we try to differentiate the country from the political regime.

Yugoslavia had a chance that has not been taken for many reasons. We doubt that history will ever again give us this chance, or rather, that we, the south Slavic peoples, will ever give it to ourselves. There were just too many tears shed in this country, too much suffering. Will we be able to make amends for it, and in what measure? Will we be able to muster the strength to face ourselves and others, to confess and repent, to forgive slowly, carefully, as we should have done before or after the World War II?

We don't wish the story of Yugoslavia falling apart to be seen as us trying to avoid our sense of responsibility from our Serbian identity. We simply wanted to share those experiences, since they are so important to us. And we feel like responsibility comes more naturally when there are memories of something that was nice and good, and not only of conflicts and hatred supported by nationalistic ideologies.

Social trauma of conflicts and wars destroys beauty and goodness, equality and humanity in general. Individuals, groups and societies are no longer subjects of social life, but its objects. There is no equality between a human subject and an object, a thing. Those who are helpless and in trauma are treated worse than slaves or "objects that talk" (*instrumenta vocalia*) were in the past. Where there are no rights and no justice, according to Aristotle, "a man can become the most devious and wild creature worse of all …"

Foulkes (1975) wrote, "… The atmosphere created in therapeutic groups must allow for the experience of helplessness, hopelessness and despair in safety…." How often are the feelings related to trauma discussed in the safety of our small analytic groups? Our experience, as well as the experience of some of the colleagues we discussed this with is, at first glance, strange. To wit, in the "safety of a small analytic group" in the last couple of years, there hasn't been much sharing of emotions related to the traumatic events our society was going through. If among the members there was someone who was directly traumatized (a refugee or someone who lost a family member in bombing or in the war), and who shared their experiences, they rarely do so again. Members generally talk freely and ask others about the most intimate details of their lives, about their weaknesses and vulnerabilities, various stressful events and losses and their anger toward current state and political organizations and the government. But about wars, bombing, isolation, accusations of the international community, guilt, shame or injustice, we mostly stay silent. We often fantasize that in the group matrix there is a Pompei where all these feelings stand petrified. However, when they participate in other social activities they mention in our group, those same members talk about their traumas. Or rather, they discuss them. When we invite them to talk about their feelings, someone mentions shame, fear of the bombings, someone mentions guilt, or injustice, but it seems as though they somehow get stuck, expecting a resolution and, sensing there isn't one, they give up. We are under the impression that this general silence is present in the community as well. Traumatized societies are like groups (Hopper, 1997). Even today, more than 20 years after the bombing, our country does not know the exact number of civilians killed, but estimates range from 800 to 2,500 adults and children. Until recently, there haven't been any projects to study the effect of depleted uranium from the bombs on the health of the population. Italy has already carried out similar research regarding their soldiers who served in these parts as members of an international peace corps, and established a larger percent of malignant and other diseases among this population. Our military headquarters has been left in ruins for over 20 years in downtown Belgrade. Just like there is no care for our own victims, there are also no public activities regarding the responsibility for the crimes Serbia has been accused of, with the exception of several apologies of politicians from Serbia and fulfillment of our obligations toward the Hague Tribunal. For example, the mass grave of Albanian victims on the outskirts of Belgrade is still left unmarked. There can be many reasons for this silence—from the fact that the traumatic period has never truly ended (negotiations about Kosovo are currently under way, there are occasional violent incidents to this day), to the general moral paralysis of the society and individuals. Populist leaders, particularly the right-oriented ones, still find it easiest to collect political points by stirring up international hatred and creating the feeling of indirect danger of new conflicts.

In a traumatized society, psycho-social space, inner and outer, is greatly radicalized, and splitting is deepened by profound anxieties (like the military headquarters building, half destroyed by bombs and half whole, still standing today). Among the citizens, the question of Serbia's responsibility varies between two extremes: some accept responsibility and all the guilt and make it even greater (we have personally heard statements such as: "We cheered for each bomb, too bad they didn't raze us to the ground."). At the same time, others are bitter and ready to give us full amnesty from any guilt and responsibility, justifying it with all the injustice and crimes of which we were victims throughout history ("Serbs are the greatest historical victims in Europe."). Both of these extreme positions are trying to present themselves as morally superior. However, we are under the impression that some of the citizens managed to avoid extremes and are currently searching for the truth, burdened by feelings of helplessness, shame, injustice, but prepared for reality and responsibility. From them we can hear their sentiment that we "have blood on our hands and can't just wash it off like Pontius Pilate." It is painful, but we must accept it, because that is the only way to make sure it never happens again. However, some people do not believe that everything is Serbia's fault, but they feel shame for what has been done. Others find Milošević guilty of everything and believe he should have also been held responsible for the damage he'd done to the citizens of

Serbia, in addition to being responsible for the wars in former republics of the Socialist Federal Republic of Yugoslavia.

There are also those who try to focus exclusively on the demanding everyday life in the country with its bad social and economic conditions. Many of them are apathetic. “Is there even a way to protect ourselves from anything, not only the bombs or, like in the dream, the rain?” It is as if the question from the dream still lingers in our reality.

We are under the impression that often in our conversations on various occasions there is something that could at first glance seem confusing: we discuss political issues like moral issues, and when we talk about ethics, politics also finds a way into that conversation. Essentially, it’s difficult for us to understand the connection between the two. Aristotle used to say that politics should be a public practice of ethics, while ethics are a social philosophy from which standards of political actions are drawn. That would be the way to avoid wars, crimes and deaths. Politics that lead into war, aggression, crime, are deeply unethical. It could be said that social trauma is above all else a question of ethics.

“… To say that we live in the social world is also to say that we live in a moral universe; to say that the psyche is patterned by power relations is to grant that it is constituted by a profound sense of … ethics” (Dalal, 2012). These statements about ethics are deeply connected to our group analytic sensibility.

Maybe we would not be exaggerating if we say that, for us, the group-analytic identity is, naturally, thinking about moral aspects of responsibility, especially in situations of social trauma.

Karl Jaspers wrote about legal, political, moral and metaphysical guilt. Legal guilt is established by a court, political responsibility by the winner. For moral guilt, the higher instance is conscience, and for the metaphysical one, it is the god. Only political responsibility is collective, in the sense that all citizens, by voting or not voting, are responsible for everything their government is doing in their name. Feelings of guilt and moral responsibility is, according to him, a personal issue. Jaspers himself also talked about how difficult it is to separate the political responsibility of a citizen from the feeling of moral responsibility as a member of the society marked as politically responsible for the war. Political responsibility is imposed by the winner, i.e., the stronger side, and that is something we could discuss. However, belonging to a family or social community whose members have committed a crime still deeply affects us.

In spite of the fact that we don’t feel personally guilty for the wars, the fact that we decided to stay here makes us responsible for the situation in our society today, and in a way responsible for everything that was done in “our name” in those wars. Responsibility carries the task to do everything possible to prevent something destructive from happening again, and to make peace a possibility.

What does it really mean to accept responsibility for what the government is doing in our name? In the moral world there is a connection between what we say and what we do. What is it that we as citizens with civil and democratic identity, and we, group analysts with our group-analytic identity, could do when it comes to the responsibility we are accepting? To vote for politics that at the given moment seem ethical, to participate in demonstrations against a non-democratic and unethical political party? (Many of the citizens of Serbia have been doing precisely this from 1991 until the fall of Milošević in 2000). Is this all we can do, and is it enough? It doesn't seem to be. In essence, some organizations have engaged socially, as non-governmental organizations (NGOs), and in cooperation with political organizations they organize various civil activities and even demonstrations. In some way, that is their job. Do we, from our group-analytic identity, have a certain special task? Once again, we are facing a challenge. We would love to ask one of our group-analytic parents what to do (in the dream, group analyst Malcolm Pines is on the phone). Does the sentence from the dream, "I think that I most of all carry the fear of whether everything will be all right," refer to us, group analysts, in this society?

We recall our professional experience and knowledge. Responsibility doesn't only lie in social and political fight against non-democratic and unjust regimes, but also in giving people a chance to work on themselves. Doesn't an analytic group with its culture and principles of ethics, truthfulness, modesty and equality of all its different members represent an important contribution to the society and its humanity? Of course, it does, and we can call ourselves really lucky to have a chance to give our contribution. If we cannot exert our influence over various "anti-groups," we can help strengthen the principles and culture of the group, in small, persistent steps.

In his essay "Collective Guilt?," Bernhard Schlink (2013), writer and professor of Law at Humboldt University, reminds us perhaps of how our group-analyst practice is an important and responsible social activity, saying:

> There is no judge, no legal proceeding or conviction that can set one free from the curse that the parents' guilt becomes for their children. *(We would add: or free the parent-victims from the feeling of helplessness and enormous suffering)* .... With each new generation, a collectively experienced historical event becomes individual and psychological, and the task of releasing a specific, historical guilt (*or, we would add, the task of giving reparation for the losses and deaths*) merges with the task of finding its own identity, which every generation has to face ...

Our help in these processes is necessary, ethical and responsible.

And maybe it will turn out that each Pompei in the group matrix is some type of shelter for emotions that fell into a catatonic state (catatonic stupor), and they will only come out of it once they find the right words within the group. We, group analysts, are in search of those words.

Joining the group-analytic community and developing our group-analytic identity in the times of difficult social traumas has opened numerous questions we felt the need to address in order to preserve within us the meaning of group analysis and our social identity in general. We faced the anti-group, we faced trauma, we experienced the idealization of the group, de-idealization, apathy and enthusiasm, desire to comprehend the incomprehensible human nature ... to finally find some inner peace in trust and faith in the group. This trust, which was shaken and traumatized, turned out to be, we shall hope, more realistic than before, and we believe that, through our work, we are going to give our contribution to the group in its dramatic dance (a balancing act) with the anti-group, even in our society today.

References

Dalal, Farhad, Specialists without Spirit, Sensualists without Heart: Psychotherapy as a Moral Endeavour. Group Analysis 45(4):405–429, 2012.

Foulkes, S. H., *Group-analytic Psychotherapy: Method and Principles*, Gordon&Breach, London, 1975.

Hopper, Earl, Traumatic Experience in the Unconscious Life of Groups: A Fourth Basic Assumption. Group Analysis 30(4):439–470, 1997.

Nitsun, Morris, *The Anti-group: Destructive Forces in the Group and Their Creative Potential*, New York: Psychology Press, 1996.

Chapter 6

Experience of Large Group at the National Congress of Serbian Psychotherapists

Snezana Kecojević Miljević, Vida Rakić Glišić, and Jelica Satarić

S.H. Foulkes and the Problem of Large Groups

During his service in the military hospital in Northfield in World War II, psychoanalyst H. Foulkes indirectly experienced a sense that large groups might be representational of a larger context like a whole hospital (Northfield), although neither then nor later was Foulkes actually in the role of the leader of a large group. Later, as a member, he participated in large groups in group-analytic symposiums and undoubtedly had a great interest in the experience of his colleagues in this field. He was a careful observer of similar activities in large groups during his visits to hospitals and therapeutic communities. As he himself wrote, he considered that large groups a welcome (1948) addendum to his other work.

At the time when I worked in a center for outpatient hospitalization of mentally ill patients, Clinical Centre (KBC), Dr. Dragiša Mišović-Dedinje, my colleague, and I organized work in our department on group-analytical principles and organized different therapeutic groups with diverse purposes. At one time, we talked a lot about the possibility of establishing a large group. Our understanding and a commonly shared knowledge is that all our groups are first born in our minds and only later become vivid in created or existing external reality. At the same time, in a kind of parallel process, we saw confirmation that the large group was present in the matrix of our team of medical staff and patient. One of our patients in a class of art therapy drew a picture of large group and how he experienced the possibility to make our small and middle therapeutic groups much larger (Figure 6.1).

Just as an individual cannot be understood outside of the context of another, so neither can the group process be understood outside of its relations with other groups or out of the context and conditions in which it exists. We cannot isolate the psychological life of the individual from biological, social, cultural or economic factors, because "it is a kind of expression of all these factors", wrote Foulkes. Factors that are horizontally linked in the current reality and also vertically integrated with the

DOI: 10.4324/9781003269649-9

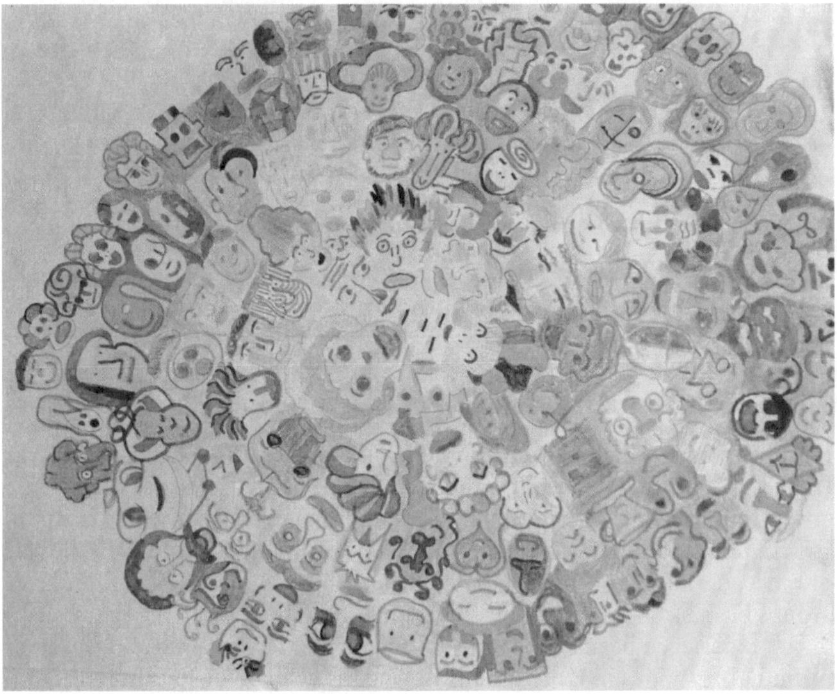

Figure 6.1 Large group painted in art therapy by a patient.

past and previous heritage. For Foulkes, "the essential difference between group and individual psychodynamic processes is negligible, almost insignificant.as it only exists when it is obtained by the virtual process of abstraction." A groups well as an individual are unique and inseparable entities, which can alternately be the focus of our observations or interest, but even then they always represent "two sides of the same coin." Therefore, small groups and their context and conditions of existence, are inseparable identities and can alternately be a focus of our observations while being "two sides of the coin."

An Experiential Large Analytical Group at the Congress of the Serbian Psychotherapist Union

A large analytical group is held every year during the Serbian SDPT (International Congress of Serbian Association of Psychotherapists) Congress, organised by group analysts from Serbia, and last year also from Bosnia and Herzegovina. The congress lasts for three days, and the large group takes place at the end of the day in two consecutive days. Last year, the Congress assembled around 300 participants mainly psychotherapists of different modalities. More than 50 people participated in the large group. The number of members varied, but it seems that around one-fifth of the congress members participated in the large group. Although it is subjected to the rules of the Large Group, this group by dint of many of its characteristics, resembles an "Impossible Group" (Weinberg, 2016), This group modality is established in the conditions of "leaking containers" i.e. diverse and varying members; some members without any group therapy experience; hosts from two different Group Analysis associations; and on top organizers who are skeptical and suspicious). The unreliability of setting boundaries from the very start could not guarantee the safety of the participants (and neither the hosts') and therefore, the guaranteed minimal conditions for possible progress were no given. However, a significant development and growth started to be noticed from the material we presented. In spite of the unreliable conditions in which this group continued, the "relaxation of censorship, disclosure of personal feelings toward other members of the group "active membership" (Foulkes, 1948) became achievable. Self-discovery was one of the minimal conditions for progress and this group worked as a powerful helping tool, facilitating the growth of the group cohesion, which is one of the key therapeutic factors that contributes to the positive therapy outcome (I.D. Yalom and M. Leszcz, 2005). The group, whose material we presented, was led by five group analysts of our Group Analytic Society Belgrade (DGAB). A few months before the congress, we lost our college, which was an important part of the organizations board of the congress and SDPT Association. We present information on this large group because of the valuable experience of establishing the distinctive cohesiveness, the reflective field and the situation of the large group. All its qualities of warmth, excitement, self-discovery, willingness to be together and share in the loss, the cathartic experience and mutual emotional exchange, resembles a small analytical group that mourns over the loss of its member.

The theme of loss "here and now" is inevitably linked with the experience of loss not only of individual members, but also with the collective experience of loss and trauma at the level of society as a whole. It is as if the further group process could go in two directions: first, in the direction of reparation of loss, namely social loss, and hope within the integration, creativity and self-esteem as a group, collectively; or it could go in the direction of regression to the unhealed experiences of traumatic disintegration, helplessness, passivity and silently waiting for a final end. Of course these processes are not alternative, in terms of "either this or that," but can merge and radiate hope and optimism in one moment and then disappear into the shadow of helplessness and hopelessness in another.

What happened next in the group?

Foulkes (1948) distinguishes three types of large groups: a problem directed large group, an experiential large group and a therapy-directed large group. In this example, the large experiential group becomes a problem-centered group.

The raised feelings of a "personal" loss of one of us and the "authentic process of grief" was transferred onto the second group but transformed into a group sliding into a schizo-paranoid position of fear of disintegration, destruction, annihilation, sickness and death. This happened through the "storytelling" of a young man in a moral tale "Ridgebeard" story about man who loses bit by bit part of his body with a sense of "no harm done" until only his heart remains. In the end, he also loses the heart and still claims "no harm done."

The impression is that through the communication of group leaders after the congress, the power of unrefined feelings and experiences over the years of virtually continuous social trauma was reflected. It was, as if we tried to somehow pour a little bit of hope into our social matrix through which memories of so many destructive events would flow. It became even clearer to us what the responsibility of our professional community was to the society as a whole. For no it does not find enough ways to help its members to move toward a process of reparation and hope.

In the days after this group session, the hosts of the group started an e-mail correspondence. In an intense exchange and back and forth discussions of the various hosts and by sharing their dreams and associations important and relevant content of the group processes emerged.

Dreams with a content of decomposing and breaking-up bodies were related to the former socialist republic, the redrawing of its borders and the loss of territory. Dreams of inflamation and burning of the mouth; dreams of unexplainable and unimaginable violence; the torching of the mouth of a police officer; dreams of jars with poison that cause death, and the name "deep forest" somewhere in a dream. Terrifying images of a yellow house, organ trafficking, bombing with depleted uranium! A glass cage for smokers associated to cancerphobia, condemned to isolation, dying by asphyxia, the quietness and paralysis while calmly waiting for the extermination.

Are we all doomed to silence, without being able to object and without acting to stop anything from happening? Did we fall for the conviction that there is no salvation, or are we in denial? The only possible exit appears to be to help one another with the utmost dedication, to open our eyes and to see! The less we suppress, deny, and deceive our- selves, the greater aur chance for a cure from mortal deceases—This was the conclusion and interpretation arrived at by this forum post festum.

From the very beginning, the large group became precious space in the matrix of the congress. A program called "The Power of Psychotherapy" was planned after the opening ceremony of the congress. It was a traditional meeting, a so-called circle of psychotherapists, which suddenly received the subtitle: "discussion by the principle of large groups." The large group setting, the arrangement of chairs by the decision of its leaders, was also changed from a large egg-cavernous circle to spirally arranged chairs with three rows. From the very beginning, the group showed great tension with attacks on group borders, leaders and setting: the key question was who decided to organize the chairs this way, who has the power to decide about changes in everyone's name? Anger was expressed—resistance toward the "insertion into change," the need for the group to become leaderless, the idea for everyone to take a chair and sit where they want, that leaders are incapable of protecting the group! All this as an impulse to do something concrete. The leaders' reminding the group that the SDPT Association changed its name to the Association of Serbian Psychotherapists (SPS) ("society" got lost in the name, and we got only SPS, the same shortcut as for Serbian Socialist Party) shifted the tension from the leaders to the organizers, and opened dialogue for a short period. The attacks and devaluations continued and statements were made that the large group is, in general, a valuable site for experience and learning but only when led "masterfully and brilliantly" like the ones from abroad. Suggestions come that a new "middle group" might be made that would be led differently and was more adapted to the needs of participants.

In a post-festum correspondence in the mini online forum of the group's leaders, impressions of great pressure and attacks on the large group were exchanged. These attacks were primarily directed at leaders, from both inside and out, about the need to set up new centers of power and decision making, to the need for new rules, to establish "the other" large group, which all together led to the final impression about the large group's values and the need to find a better way of making it think. But all the discomfort from the pressure of uncertainty with which the leaders battled, whether the boundaries of the group will be penetrated and the unimaginable chaos of the crowd overwhelmed it from within, symbolically was dreamed about by a leader of the group. She shared the dream in which her apartment is rented to another person by tricking her, and her frantic efforts to, with the help of a tiny key, restrain the new residents from violently getting inside. The rest of the facilitators wrestled with feelings and impressions of the attack on all sorts of precious items through devaluation. Group members were musing about the former Serbian province of Kosovo which they felt. should be given away since it was no longer Serbian. Similar trends could be constructed and detected in the large group. Unexpected attacks, a sense of treasons by our colleagues in moments of greatest vulnerability. We were reminded that our countries history is littered with treason, fratricide and parricide, The large group, it was suggested, would be "masterfully and brilliantly" led by the group leaders from abroad! We were told that attacks were to be withstood at all costs. Again a reminder that he battle for Košare lasted more than a month, where the enemies silently faced each other, constantly threatening each other.

The pressure was similar in the large group in which the leaders battled with the group, whether by holding the boundaries of the large group or by trying to avoid an unimaginable chaos of the group members which would penetrate and overwhelm the group from within. There appeared to be an inability to be in the here and now and the need to fly away or reach into a distant future was the only thing that promised salvation.

Bridges, Walls, Spaces

"Only a certain number of individuals in their emotional development reach something which could be called the status of the whole," wrote D. Winnicott, (1969). In the same article, titled "Berlin Walls," Winnicott wrote about the Berlin Wall as a phenomenon that can be found everywhere in the world, pointing to the paradox of the phenomenon in which, he said, humanity has accomplished some sort of unity.

Comparing today's world with that of 1969 as described by Winnicott, we would say that today, the world is far away from his idealized image and from the achievement of "oneness" despite the powerful modern electronic ways of connecting and communication. Even though the Berlin Wall was demolished more than two decades ago, the idea of new walls is not disappearing.

Terzijski Bridge dates from the early 13th century and is built between the Serbian and Albanian villages of Kosovo and Metohia on a river with two names: Ribnik (Albanian) and Erenik (Serbian). The bridge enables both connection and boundaries between the two sides as the line of military peace. However, the bridge is very old and out of use, so the river is the division line that postpones the conflict and separates the opposing sides.

Successful and full integration leads to the depressive position in which a person bears a potential state of war using one internal "Berlin Wall," a line of military peace that, in the worst case, only postpones conflict and in the best case separates the opposing sides, enabling the parts freed from conflict to continue with the "art of peace." In the space of "in between" where the truce rules, and in the shadows of the Berlin Wall or on the Terzijski Bridge (which was built right on the point at which if there was no wall, or river, there would be war), the art of peace may be practiced and the boundaries that separate can be crossed over without consequence. "If a farmer while plowing his field, can't play with the border by crossing it back and forth" (or by crossing the bridge), "then we know that the state of potential war exists in that area, so we don't search for the art of peace at that place nor for the playful creativity" (D. Winnicott, 1969). (Berlin Wall history is also a tragic history of many individuals who perished while illegally crossing it.)

In the large group "in between space "(M. Pines) are spaces in which playfulness and creativity become possible. This becomes possible by baring the antagonism between all large group-members as well as their differences and diversities. The group diversity can originate from different schools and models of psychotherapy as mentioned at the beginning of this chapter. Without denying the antagonism and difference amongst them, the group becomes productive in a positive way. It does not need to resort to pushing the limit and dominate the weaker social group or withdraw into schizoid isolation.

Conclusion

The reflective space spread out from this actual large group situation as an echo that associated and moved us toward the interpretive work and processing. In the new online forum, among the hosts of large group, one extension of "in between" reflective space (M. Pines) was created in which we could continue the dialogue as to further process, associate, connect, and integrate through this reflective echo of group dynamic (Maré 1972a; Maré 1972). The strength of this established matrix of the large group demonstrated its power and the presented authentic self-discovery, which achieved group cohesion, reliable bounds, and not complete but significant safety (Foulkes, 1948), made the minimal possible conditions for the group subsistence and development.

References

Bion, W.R., Experiences in Groups and Other Papers. London: Tavistock Publications Limited, 1961.

de Maré, P., Large group psychotherapy: a suggested technique. Group Analysis. 5, 106–108, 1972a.

de Maré, Patrick, Large Group perspectives, Spheres of Group Analysis, pp.45–50, ed. by T.E. Lear, Group Analytic Society Publication, 1972b.

Foulkes, S.H., Therapeutic Group Analysis. Maresfield Library, Karnac Classics, London, 1984.

Foulkes, S.H., Introduction to Group Analytic Psychotherapy, William Heinemann Medical Books Ltd., 1948, reprinted by Karnac Books, London, 2005.

Foulkes, S.H., Selected Papers of S.H. Foulkes Psychoanalysis and Group Analysis. Karnac Books, London, 1990.

Jones, Maxwell, The therapeutic Community: A New Treatment Method in Psychiatry. Basic Books, 1953.

Kreeger, Lionel C., The Large Group: Dynamics and Therapy. Routledge, London, 1975.

Le Bon G., The Crowd: A Study of the Popular Mind, 1986.

Le Bon, G., Psihologija gomile. Delfi, 2007.

Lipgar, R.M., Malcom, P., Building on Bion: Branches. Contemporary Development and Application of Bion's Contributions of Theory and Practice. Jessica Kingsly Publishers, London, NY, 2003.

Main, Thomas, The Hospital as a Therapeutic Institution. Bulletin of the Menninger Clinic, 10, 66–70, 1946.

Schneider, S., Weinberg, H., The Large Group-Revisited: The Herd, Primal Horde, Crowds and Masses. Jessica Kingsley Publishers, 2003.

Stein, M.S., Stein, J., Malcom Pines, London. Psychotherapy in Practice: A Life in the Mind. Butterworth-Heinemann, Oxford, 2000.

Turquet, P., 'Threats to identity in the large group.' In L. Kreeger (ed) The Large Group: Dynamics and Therapy. Constable, London, 1975.

Varvarin, Volkan, Štajner-Popović, Kadvila, Vučo, Fonda. Psihoanaliza i rat, Čigoja štampa, 2001.

Weinberg, H., Impossible Groups that Flourish in Leaking Container. Challenging Analytical Theory. 40th Annual GASI, 2016.

Winnicott, D.W., The Berlin Walls in Frojd, Anštajn, Glover, Moni-Kerli, Vinikot, 1969.

Yalom, I.D., Leszcz, M., The Theory and Practice of Group Psychotherapy, 5th ed. Basic Books, New York, 2005.

Part III

Social Trauma in the Consulting Room

Chapter 7

The Echoes of Social Trauma in the Consulting Room

Ivanka Dunjić

> "I am alone in a dark wood and I am scared. Then I meet a girl in partisan uniform, she takes me by the hand and leads me to a nice clearing. She then disappears and I am alone and scared again. And all of a sudden, here comes Tito on a beautiful white horse. He bends over me, with a warm smile, and says 'There is going to be a war and this country will be destroyed. But don't you worry, everything will be fine in the end.'"

This dream was told to me some months ago in a session, by Ana, an over-anxious middle-aged lady, as an illustration of her premonitory capacities. It was dreamt a long time ago, in the mid-1980s, when she was 8 years old, then it was forgotten and remembered again in the 1990s, when the war started. Intelligent and professionally successful, privately she was stuck for years, unable to make life decisions, to get married or to have children, all the time paralyzed and unable to make a distinction between her anxious expectations and premonitions. This culminated in panic attacks with the anxiety of getting mad.

Where did this "premonitory" knowledge come from? Was it an intuitive knowledge from social unconscious or knowledge drawn from her foundational and family matrices, transferred across generations. Were her fears of a future breakdown from something that had already happened in the past, as British psychoanalyst, Donald Winnicott would say? I remember that I immediately reacted to her dream with an uncanny filling of connectedness and deep understanding. Having no associations herself, she was asked about that period of her life, and she recalled the unhappy years of her childhood and adolescence when she was suffering from school phobia, never belonging to peer groups, having just one best friend and running away from all social situations, desperately hiding behind false health excuses. Slightly guided by my questions, some topics related to the history of her family were opened. It came out that her grandparents actively belonged to different sides in the civil war during the World War II. Those on her paternal side were loyal to the king and those on her maternal side were partisans and communists. People loyal to the king in the postwar

DOI: 10.4324/9781003269649-11

history were labelled as traitors. Two families never really connected, and from her early days, she was exposed to hostile messages that they were exchanged via their granddaughter as well as to her parents' lifelong quarrels, all while keeping a formal appearance of harmony. She was emotionally much closer to her paternal grandmother, but she was struggling with problems of taking sides and loyalty all the time.

The years when Ana was at school coincided with the years after Tito's death, when he was even more celebrated and idealized than when was alive. We were surrounded with political slogans "AFTER TITO—TITO" and "TITO IS ALIVE," having instead of a new president a bizarre creation, called "collective presidency" made up of representatives of all the republics. With the "après coup" knowledge we could say that it reflected the fragility of the Yugoslav foundation matrix, torn between tensions and mutual distrust, and full of futile and grotesque efforts to glue it up by idealizing the dead leader. We all know what the outcome was. Following that line of thought, we could imagine that Ana's dream could have been dreamt by almost any citizen of this country (I guess that explains my instant familiar reaction to it). Its rhythmic repetition of scary and confronting elements could reflect the rhythm of war and peace, massive social traumas and abrupt political changes interrupted with short periods of hope and serenity. We could also connect that with compulsively repeated collective search for an idealized political leader-saviour, as well as with the lack of possibility to learn from recent tragic experiences. I will illustrate that with some facts: for elderly citizens, when the war started in the 1990s, it was the fifth war in their lifetime; they had survived two Balkan wars in 1912 and 1913 and two World Wars. They could also say that they had lived in seven different countries, without moving geographically from the place where they were born: Kingdom of Serbia, Kingdom of Serbs, Croats and Slovenes, Federal People's Republic of Yugoslavia, Socialist Federal Republic of Yugoslavia, Federal Republic of Yugoslavia, the Republic of Serbia and Montenegro, and now (finally?) the Republic of Serbia.

Coming back to the consulting room with Ana, we could imagine that her difficulties in socializing were connected with the fact that her fragile social identity was suffused with family political conflict. In the "here and now" of our relationship, obviously, the help of the partisan girl as a fellow traveller was not reassuring enough at the beginning. She needed me to be a much stronger, omnipotent figure, a "subject supposed to know," so she used to take a little notebook and write down some very ordinary things that I would say as ultimate wisdoms. Some difficulties in Ana's world could be connected to her social unconscious, as German-British psychiatrist and psychoanalyst S. H. Foulkes defined it—an "... internalized social world of which people were unaware, and also the properties of external social world of which people were unaware." Foulkes also said that an "individual is as much compelled and moulded by those colossal forces as by his own id" (Hopper and Weinberg 2011).

While preparing for this chapter and thinking about Ana, I had some interesting personal insight, emerging from the unthought known to the daylight. I was born in a family that was very disappointed with the local political outcome of World War II, so the attitude toward the communist society and its institutions was one of distrust and contempt, with nostalgia for the beautiful times before the war. Very often I would get an alternative version of the history lessons we learnt at school: "No it did not happen like that, this is how it really happened ...." So, from my early days I was introduced to postmodern realm of subjectivity, and it was not evident what the factual history was. Although growing up with the impression that I was living in a wrong society, I was doing well at school and I was very interpersonally connected in terms of friendships and peer groups, but completely disconnected and alienated from any social, political or institutional engagement. Consciously, I knew that I was attracted to psychoanalysis out of fascination with the fantasy world in art and literature, and its hidden latent meanings. This time, I also realized that my choice was motivated by the defensive illusion that psychoanalysis as a chamber profession was an escape from the institutional and the social, and also a field where different realities coexist. However, this defensive illusion was not meant to last long as very soon it was interrupted by the traumatic social changes in our country. Also, almost at the same time, it was interrupted by the beginning of my group-analytic education and its metaphor of the Mobius strip (Pines) and other group-analytic concepts helpful for understanding individual/social connectedness. My whole professional life, since the time I qualified, first as an individual then as a group analyst (late 1980s and beginning of the 1990s), has been spent developing against the background of social traumata, just to mention the most dramatic ones: nationalistic, totalitarian regime, war, fragmentation of Yugoslavia, sanctions, refugees, years of demonstrations, poverty and criminalization of society, NATO bombing, democratic revolution, assassination of a prime minister and failure of democratic changes...

Social Trauma in the Consulting Room

Taking now the consulting room as our chosen context in which social traumatic events were translated by individuals or members of small therapy groups, it is quite clear that, for all those years, the social was so intrusive that it was hard to ignore it, whether it was manifested loudly, silently or it was disguised. The challenge was more how to articulate it clinically in the most helpful way (Hopper, 1996).

Acute Social Trauma—"Being in the Same Boat"

The next example I would like to share with you is about a situation of acute social trauma, its specificity being that it was connected with the fact that the therapist and the patients were sharing the same destiny, and that the inter-subjective contextualization of the social reality was inevitably affected by it.

The evening when the bombing of Belgrade started, I was conducting a small group. Two of the seven members were absent, estimating that it was not wise to leave home. The others were joking about their exaggerated anxiety. One man said that he was carrying an axe in his backpack in case we got buried under the rubble and everybody laughed. The prevailing atmosphere nurtured by gossip was that the bombing would probably be avoided this time. Fifty minutes later, we heard the air raid alert. Somebody said that it was a test, and one lady journalist said: "They have announced there will be no testing. This is it." I remember that for a second I felt paralyzing fear. Then, as all the eyes were turned to me, I knew that I had to be calm and decide what the best thing to do would be—to continue the session and do my usual work by providing some holding and containment for their anxieties (giving priority to the emotional security), or end the group and send the members home, as quickly as possible. Sincerely, at that moment, I had a strong need to get to my family and see that everybody was safe (whatever that would mean). This short-lived dilemma was resolved by a pragmatic reaction of a young woman who said that she was living at the other side of the river, and that she had better find a way to get home. Relieved, I proposed that we end the group and the members organized the transport home among themselves. I think that I have learned several important things from that unforgettable experience of "being in the same boat." First, not only that in such situations does the therapist have to carry the function of holding and containment while feeling very fragile and afraid herself, but she also has to decide quickly which reality is to be prioritized, external or internal. Second, that her usual position of giving priority to internal reality might be defensive—in the example I described, I did not decide to finish the group out of guilt for wishing to run away. Also, in such situations, more than ever, the therapist has to contain the omnipotent projections, as defences against helplessness and insecurity, sometimes colluding with patients against the common sense.

Unconscious Constraints Connected with Social Trauma

Although from time to time, during the war and several years after it, we had the opportunity to work with severely traumatized persons, usually war veterans or refugees who were displaying all known short- and long-term consequences of trauma, I would like to focus this time on other more discrete, covert and unconscious ways that social trauma can shape the lives of individuals, and also on the different ways it was actualized and articulated in the therapy process. In such cases the consulting room becomes a privileged location for exploration of inner worlds of socially traumatizing outer realities.

But before entering concrete clinical issues, I would like to make a brief review of some important questions and theoretical concepts from psychoanalysis and group analysis, in order to avoid simplifying and reducing the relationship between outer and inner realities merely to the loop of mutual interferences.

Social as belonging to historical facts

If we regard social traumata only in terms of external reality acting upon individuals, large groups and societies exploring their influence and transformation to subjective experience, we are faced with difficulties. Although we cannot deny the existence of historical facts, even in case of some recent events, it is difficult to know "what really did happen" because of complexity and all unconscious and purposeful distortions. Winnicott said that history is always propaganda. One of my patients, a history student from Bosnia, abandoned his studies after several years of desperate efforts to discover the truth about the famous Sarajevo assassination in 1914. The deeper we go into the past, the more difficult it is to make a distinction between history and inter-subjective construction of myths and phantasies forming the building blocks of social unconscious as defined by Earl Hopper and Haim Weinberg (2011). Regine Scholz (2011) points to the difference between the communicative memory relating to the events belonging to recent past events that are passed on to future generations through personal family narratives, and cultural memory connected to ancient events that would fade from memory unless they were preserved by cultural institution of societies such as books, monuments, places, and rituals (Scholz 2011, Assmann 2004).

Social-external/internal

Going further with external/internal dimension: the majority of psychoanalytic schools link the social with the external and regard social as something from the outside that enters an already formed inside (Dalal 1998), meaning that individual psychology arises somehow prior and outside of the group, and that the understanding of the individual is the basis for understanding of the group and the social. The external/internal interact through processes of introjection and projection, and by introjection the social is established in the internal world. "People internalize their social world, and much has been projecting in them ..." (Dalal 1998). For example, the Freudian notion of superego is a representation of internalized and trans-generationally transmitted prohibitions. Not only is the social at the same time internal and external, but for some schools, represented by what Dalal called "radical," S. H. Foulkes, Norbert Elias and Farhad

Dalal himself, the social is prior to the individual, the unconscious is structured by the social, which is expressed in the phrase "the social as unconscious." Extending Foulkes's stance about the group and the individual being abstractions, and paraphrasing Winnicott, Dalal says that there is no individual outside society, ideology or discourse. Structuring processes of ideology and discourse are instituted in social unconscious, swallowed by language. Those impersonal structures that are swallowed by language represent the indigested pieces of society (Dalal 1998).

Relation of social trauma to social unconscious

Even a superficial look at the tensions on the international scene suggests that living with continuous social traumata is not just a Serbian specialty. We are witnessing local wars in different parts of the world, September 11th and other terrorist's attacks with many victims, global economy crisis, ecology warnings, Brexit, immigrant crisis, awakening of extreme right movements, mentioning of a World War III in connection of the worsening relationship between Russia and the USA and so on. Then, if we follow the historical line, we could say that we are all children or grandchildren of World War II—victims or survivors, that we have grown up in the atmosphere of the Cold War and nuclear threat, many of us in totalitarian societies and in the shadow of horrible pictures of Holocaust and Hiroshima. Does it mean that social unconscious of all contemporary European citizens is rooted in a deeply traumatized foundation matrix? Or even wider, that social unconscious, is always related to traumatic collective experiences? Both, Earl Hopper and Haim Weinberg, although disagreeing upon definition, are in agreement about traumatic essence of social unconscious and defences against awareness of painful helplessness: "Primal internalization processes are always colored by traumatic experience of loss, separation and failed dependency and are predisposing factors in secondary internalization of collective memories of social trauma … (and) …helplessness and traumatic experience are at the heart of human condition" (Hopper & Weinberg, 2011, p. xxxix).

Hopper (1996) designed a paradigm, illustrating the four possibilities concerning the presence or absence of patients' preoccupation with social and political topics and the consequent analyst's focus on internal or external reality. He argues that although from the point of view of classical psychoanalysis the analyst's interventions focused on external, political and social would be considered as problematic, defensive and collusive … "It is equally defensive and collusive not to discuss social and political facts and to avoid anxiety about them by turning to the more familiar concerns and concepts."

I remember that during the bombing, with the exception of this first evening, I felt most secure when working with patients. All of them who stayed in the country, kept coming as usual and we only moved the time of the sessions to the morning hours due to the probability of air raid alerts. Partly, I suppose, that for both sides there was some defensive collusion in the phantasy that as far as the setting was preserved, our lives were not in danger, but also that it was a manifestation of resiliency. When you live in a long-lasting socially traumatic situation, with no visible end, you have to reestablish the meaning of more private and internal issues. Also remember that during those months, we had weekly meetings of our psychoanalytic society, with excellent attendance and most interesting discussions. One of our colleagues used to call them "Titanic orchestra."

In the same article, Hopper proposes to change Malan's therapeutic triangle of space and time dimensions into a therapeutic square, including the dimension of the social unconscious. He says that although *here and now* is a privileged "hot" focus for different psychoanalytic schools because of transference enactment of most important unconscious issues, the social unconscious could be as deep as so-called Freudian unconscious, and covertly present in all space and time dimensions of therapy. Also, sometimes the reconstruction of *there and then*, with the extension from personal past to previous generations could be of crucial curative importance. In the example of Ana, the constraints of social unconscious were recognizable in the here and now of transference, and in all aspects of her past and present life.

It is also interesting to see the manifestations of social unconscious in the here and now of small groups in the form of totalitarian objects emerging from the foundation matrix.

From time to time, a person in the group says, "We do not talk politics here …" followed by silent agreement of others, without awareness that by this very sentence the politics has already been introduced in the form of totalitarian censorship. Or similarly: "It is forbidden to talk to each other outside the group." On such an occasion, we can see how totalitarian ideology is infiltrated in a democratic group-analytic culture, and how very often recommendations are perverted into strict rules.

Luka and the Independence of Kosovo

One Sunday afternoon in winter 2004, the independence of Kosovo was declared and the new republic was immediately recognized by several countries. Although not a surprise, this event provoked strong political tensions and reactions on internal and international scenes, as well as intense and mixed feelings among Serbian citizens that could be summarized around fears of a new war crisis and fragmentation of the country and the resignation about being unfairly treated by the international community. Demonstrations were organized in different towns with paradoxical results: the rage was expressed against town property, there were four dead and many wounded.

Interestingly, this topic was almost absent from Monday sessions, and I also forgot it, as for me it meant another disappointment with institutions and violation of procedures. Then came Luka, who brought his last night's dream: He is driving his special favourite car and he comes to the state border. There is a friendly policeman, who does not ask to check his passport but instead gives him the sign to pass and greats him with traditional tree-finger salute. Luka notices that those tree fingers are cut off. No associations. "What a stupid dream. The dreams generally are stupid, no use!" This was Luka's well-known attitude toward dreams as well as toward other mental contents. He was a young physician, with a macho attitude, preoccupied with his body and the fear of sudden death. He came to therapy, pressed by his wife, only after detailed medical exams had confirmed his perfect health. The only meaningful link that he was able to make between his symptoms and his life, was the birth of his son and a thought that flashed through his head when he saw the baby for the first time: "He is so fragile, now I must be strong and stay alive, to protect him." The same day he had his first panic attack and thought that he was dying. Probably under the impression of yesterday's events, but also because of the presence of elements such as frontier, Serbian three-finger national salute with rich symbolism, ambiguous meanings, and castrated policeman (official authority), I suggested that his dream was maybe connected to yesterday's Kosovo events. He replied: "I could not care less about those things, I never watch TV" … and he continued to talk about the car from the dream, an old timer that he wished to buy, but his wife was against it. His refusal was so intense that for a moment I felt that my proposition was totally inadequate, as if we were not a part of the same reality. I was even more surprised when some weeks later, he casually mentioned that both his parents were Serbs with Kosovo origin. Luka soon left therapy. He got rid of his anxiety by sticking to manic defences (as announced in his dream—no passport, no boundary, castrated super ego figure), choosing to lead an exciting promiscuous life. In retrospect, we can suppose that Luka's fragile masculine identity was based on narcissistic identification with his rich and powerful father and unresolved Oedipal issues. Internally, he was not ready to be the father to his baby son, and in the same way he was not able to deal with new social events that threatened his narcissistic balance with humiliating castration. His dream could thus be seen as a creation of his social unconscious, represented vividly by symbolic and iconic means … "social forces of which he was unaware" (Foulkes 1964). My associations to actual social context were left to hang in the air, with no possibility of any meaningful inter-subjective co-construction. Does this clinical example offer any useful ways of understanding what was happening on the level of society, with Luka as a spokesperson? If we assume the existence of isomorphism between a traumatized individual and a traumatized society, it is tempting to use Luka's dream as a picture of collective unconscious phantasy in which the loss of a part of the territory is equated with the threat of castration and humiliation, together with manic defences against it. The tree-finger salute was used in Serbian history at the beginning of the 19th century among the rebels against Turks signifying the Holy trinity, then rediscovered by Serbian opposition leaders in the 1990s. It could also be very tempting and easy to connect Vamik Volkan's chosen trauma (Volkan 2006), elaborated on the example of Kosovo battle (14th century), and actual political tensions about Kosovo, but it would be too simplified. I tend to agree with Regine Scholz that events belonging to a very distant past are transmitted by cultural, not communicative memory, and can be abused by the propaganda and the media, as "empty signifiers" in service of actual political needs. Much more recent traumas, belonging to World War I and World War II that were transmitted verbally and non-verbally from generation to generation, as un-mourned losses could be actualized by new traumas.

In Tito's Yugoslavia, the imposed official politics of "unity and brotherhood" was a glue spread over the wounds of two big wars. The manifestations of national identity, especially for Serbs and Croats, as the most numerous nations, were sanctioned. The Serbian refugees from Kosovo, after World War II ended, were forbidden by special law to return to their homes, for unclear reasons. Those suppressions prevented deep reconciliation and mourning to take place, so it was easy for Milosevic to pull the skeletons out of the closet. Although the myth of Kosovo was abused by his politics, the real emotional power was coming from more recent traumas.

The next two clinical examples are meant to illustrate the idiosyncratic ways that transgenerational traumas created unconscious constraints, representing clinically important clues.

Mina and the vampires

Mina, a highly educated and urbane young woman came to therapy because of anxiety attacks that started when she moved to her fiancé's home. His parents had died some months before in a car accident. Mina could not stand the gloomy atmosphere in the house and she felt as if the ghosts of his parents were all around. She felt claustrophobic, as if caught in a horror movie, and wanted to run away all the time. At the same time, she felt guilty for not being able to be more sympathetic to her fiancé. One day she discussed a dream: She is taking a bus ride and suddenly she realizes that she is the only person alive on the bus, all other passengers are vampires … she woke up horrified. Her only association was that as a child, and even later, she had a strong fear of vampires and zombies. She used to imagine that people around her were just pretending to be alive. To my question about losses in her family, at first she denied having any and then she remembered that her grandmother, who actually raised her, lost her parents and 15 relatives in one night during the World War II. They were all taken to a concentration camp, and never returned. Always dressed in black, she was a perennial mourner (Volkan). Too many deaths to be buried and mourned, they were presented as neither dead nor alive in the unconscious of the next generations. It proved to be an important clue for the understanding of Mina's anxieties, and of her inability to empathize with her bereaved fiancé.

Sara and the September 11th

The tragic events in the USA provoked strong reactions of astonishment, fear and compassion. Everybody was talking about them, everywhere, and in almost all of the sessions as well.

In the small group the day after, this topic also took central place with an exceptional uneasiness. The anxiety could be felt in the air. The high intensity of emotions could be explained by the fact that only two years after the bombing of Serbia had passed and that fear and resentment had not been worked through yet, but also by the specific composition of that group. Four members were refugees from different parts of former Yugoslavia—two from Croatia, one from Bosnia and one from Kosovo, and three members had been born in Belgrade. The reactions were: The new World War is going to start! They are going to blame and bomb us again! There were even revengeful ones such as: Now they can see how it is when you lose everything! These met with disapproval: How can you be like that, you have to make a distinction between politics and innocent people, and the discussion was taking place between those more paranoid and radical, and those more emphatic and democratic and we could say that this was reflecting a usual split in the foundation matrix between two Serbias that emerged easily from the foundation into dynamic matrix of the group. Then suddenly, Sara burst in tears and anger; I cannot stand you, a cannot stand this disaster. You are sitting here and talking and those poor people are suffering dead and wounded, I would like to be with them. This was a surprise, because for two years in the group she was most of the time silent, expressing only conventional attitudes, supportive to others, very difficult to reach in a personal way. The only exceptions from this "low profile" attitude were her repeated nightmares of being closed in a glass box like in an aquarium, with many other people, and they were all suffocating. Up to that moment, in spite of group efforts, the dream was not connected with anything meaningful for her.

All interest from outside situation was then turned to Sara, who was also surprised by her outburst and willing to understand it, and the whole group was engaged in joint work and a creative intersubjective space was established. For the first time, she revealed to us her family secret. Her father and aunt were Jewish war orphans from parents killed in concentration camps, probably in a gas chamber. They did not like to talk about it, it was a taboo at home, and they changed their family name into a Serbian one. Her aunt became a radical antiwar activist, but her father was a withdrawn and silent man, who spent most of his time in his room, being periodically severely depressed. For Sara, he was out of reach and she longed to be closer to him, but at the same time was afraid to imagine the pain he was suffering.

Somebody from the group suggested that her dream was her imagination of a gas chamber, as a horrifying picture about what had happened to her grandparents and what was in her father's head. This session was a turning point in Sara's therapy, she found a way to be more included, lost her weight, as if she came to life.

Instead of Conclusion

Two months ago, while reading some articles about the war in Croatia and Bosnia, I was surprised by the intensity of uneasiness that I felt, almost physically. More than 25 years have passed, there was nothing new to discover. That night, I had a dream: I am with my sister in the house we used to live in the 1990s. She receives a phone call from a person with a strange name and is told that we have to shelter and help a lot of wounded people at our home, but it is very dangerous because we do not know which side they belong to and if we were caught we could be punished and shot. I remember that I felt intense fear and at the same time anxiety about our poor resources for help as we had only some bandages and alcohol from the home first aid kit. I was also angry with my sister for placing the two of us in such an impossible situation.

In the morning, while thinking about the dream, I felt that it helped me to understand the uneasy feeling from the previous day. I remembered that during the war, on a daily basis, for several years I felt the same mixture of fear and guilt, unable to find relief by taking sides. The poor supplies for help reminded me of the feeling that I sometimes have: that psychoanalysis is a poor and insufficient remedy when confronted with massive disasters, something like offering cakes to hungry people.

References

Assmann, Jan, Phylogenetisches oder kulturelles Gedächtnis - Sigmund Freud und das Problem der unbewussten Erinnerungsspuren [Phylogenetic or cultural memory - Sigmund Freud and the problem of unconscious memory traces]. Freiburger literaturpsychologische Gespräche, 23, 63–79, 2004.

Dalal, Farhad, Taking the Group Seriously: Towards a post-foulkesian group analytic theory, International Library of Group Analysis, 1998.

Foulkes, Siegmund Heinrich, *Therapeutic Group Analysis.* George Allen & Unwin, London, 1964.

Hopper, Earl & Weinberg, Haim, Introduction, in: Earl Hopper and Haim Weinberg (Eds.), The Social Unconscious in Persons, Groups and Societies - Mainly Theory (Vol. 1), pp. xxiii- lvi, Karnac Books, London, 2011.

Hopper, Earl, The Social Unconscious in clinical work: a fourth basic assumption, Group Analysis, 30, 439–470, 1996.

Scholz, Regine, The Foundation Matrix and the Social Unconscious, in: Earl Hopper and H. Weimberg, The Social Unconscious in Persons, Groups and Societies, Vol 1, Mainly Theory, 265–285, Karnac Books, London, 2011.

Volkan, Vamik, Killing in the Name of Identity: A Study of Bloody Conflicts, Pitchstone Publishing, Charlottesville, 2006.

Chapter 8

Recalling the Traumatic and Pacts of Denial in Psychoanalytic Group Psychotherapy

Klimis Navridis

The traumatic, has been the cornerstone of psychoanalysis. Approximately 40 years following its founding moment, the traumatic was furthermore connected, in Northfield, to the psychoanalytic discovery of the small group (Bion, 1961). Originally—I am referring to Breuer and Freud's findings on hysteria—the traumatic originated in repressed early childhood experiences of sexual harassment, namely, the intolerability of Love. In Northfield, it was the trauma of war on the human body and psyche that became the starting point for the psychoanalytic discovery of groups; in other words, the impenetrability and inseparability of Death.

The Traumatic as the Mental Basis of Groups

This constant tug-of-war between repetition (which is familiar) and the unfamiliar (which is represented by the new), between connection and disconnection, Love and Death, lies at the basis of the process of formation, as well as evolution, in all group situations. In other words, the mental basis of the group is none other than the traumatic. The terror of the unfamiliar, caused by the presence of others within the clinical environment of the psychoanalytic psychotherapeutic group—the exposure in their eyes, which reflects an internal threat of confronting anything within you whose existence you do not even dare suspect and the compulsory sharing with others—may, for some, be a traumatic experience of collective mental hyper-stimulation with a particularly traumatic impact (Kaës, 1993, p. 248).

It is as though the group's mental experience itself brings about a massive regression in participants and, consequently, the revival, in some of them, of repressed traumatic experiences from their childhood that unconsciously resonate with similar phantasies of the other participants. These situations, which may be traumatic even for analysts, particularly when they are novices (Grappin, 2017, p.55), lead to the "organization" of defence mechanisms of denial and *subconscious pacts of denial* (Kaës, 2009), that is, situations which in transference (and counter-transference) seem to belie what appears to be happening in the present, to reverse it,

DOI: 10.4324/9781003269649-12

shift it and dramatize it. Some participants, for whom the group becomes a particularly fearsome object, are systematically late coming to sessions or prematurely end therapy. These reactions, too, might cause trauma to some members of the group.

In such cases, these particular members, provided their psychopathology and family history supports it, might unwittingly undertake to become the *anxiety-bearers, shame-bearers* and *symptom-bearers* of an entire group (Kaës, 1994, pp. 229–230). Because there is the element of unconscious repetition, meaning that voluntarily repeating such a representation is not something new for them; these same persons did the same (e.g. in their family) and continue to do so in other group situations besides this particular group.

This game between then and now, internal and external, the subjective and the shared and collective, the real that causes pain and that into which the real is transformed in the imagination and changes, sometimes severely tests the group's and the therapist's ability to contain. In other words, they put to the test the containing ability of *psychic envelopes*[1] (Anzieu, 1985). At the same time, they assist in the mentalization and mental process and symbolization of the trauma, both at an inter-subjective and an individual level. This is because the group permits a different dramaturgical "construction" of the subjective trauma, through another story which, on the one hand, has the capacity to connect the subjects to each other, while on the other hand, by somehow removing the exclusive property of the trauma from these specific persons, transfers it to the group as an inter-subjective whole. This de-personalization and grouping of the traumatic, both the involuntary and voluntary estrangements from the individual subject who, until recently, had undertaken to bear it, at first operates as a relief, while at the same time, subsequently, paving the way to a subjectivation emancipated from trauma.

Clinical Case

The group I wish to refer to begin with a trauma and a rebuttal. At the second session, one of the members, a young woman, announces that she is facing difficulties and that for "purely financial" reasons she has decided to discontinue. She will be coming to the group only one last time. Five members remained: three women and two men. Anna, 34 years old, with a narcissistic disorder, comes from an abusive and violent family environment, and lives with a man 30 years older than herself, with whom she quarrels constantly. At first, she used to arrive late, leaving messages on my answering machine that something unexpected had turned up.

She always clutched a huge, open handbag, overflowing with boxes of medicine or cigarettes, make-up tubes, hairbrushes, bottles of water and other odds and ends. In a way, this overflowing handbag that came and went to and from the meetings seemed to metaphorically represent the group's psychic envelope (*envelope psychique*, according to Didier Anzieu (1985) and René Kaës (1979, 2007)), both in the patient herself and the other participants, as if it could not contain the group's anxiety or was in danger of bursting at any moment. She would rarely speak, but when she did, she was very direct, although she frequently ended up being dismissive or expressing threatening and revengeful wishes of leaving the group prematurely.

For example, with a derogatory comment, she attacked Eleni, another 41-year-old participant, also with a narcissistic disorder, bulimic and with an abusive family history (particularly from her mother to herself). It was one of the rare occasions that Eleni had dared to speak. She usually remained silent, complaining that she suffered from intense feelings of shame, occasionally looking in my direction, with a sneaky conspiratorial smile, as if we both secretly shared something the others shouldn't know. She had mentioned that Anna's systematic delays upset her, that she felt they were derogatory, that Anna's behaviour, and particularly in the way she would look at her, reminded her of her mother and enraged her. At first, Anna, without a word, gave her a look full of disdain and then said something that sounded most insulting. Eleni was furious and threatened that if Anna ever spoke to her again in this manner, she might even hit her.

Revival of the Traumatic

It was clear that unwittingly and without their realizing it, something very deep and traumatic was resurfacing in the group, allowing each of the two (Anna and Eleni) to be reflected in the other. There was something that simultaneously both connected and alienated them: namely, something that connected them confrontationally. At the same time, anything traumatic unconsciously corresponding to the other members appeared to have become transcribed in the fantasy scenario of this conflict. This particular episode plunged the group in its familiar sadistic silence, which for many months was the suffocating background of almost all our sessions. An anal silence of sadistic withholding, which tried the patience of the group, its members, and also my own (Wood, 2016).

Occasionally, in the unfolding of the first year's sessions, usually following violent derogatory attacks toward my person, or threats of premature discontinuation of therapy, the participants, one after the other, took the risk of making very personal and painful revelations to the group, in an atmosphere of particularly intense emotion. Although this appeared to touch upon all the others, they continued to remain silent, almost indifferent, as though they had heard nothing. What participants brought to the group were the traumatic experiences of loss, abandonment, betrayal, injustice and humiliation.

My interventions, when not appearing to fall on deaf ears, most of the time had a negative impact on the group; at times they were considered inappropriate or untimely, at other times they were found incriminating or aggressive (nor were they, possibly, entirely wrong, although I was certain of the opposite, believing they were wronging myself). During the sessions, I was frequently unbearably bored or was stifled by waves of extreme resentment or disdain for specific members, or for the entire group and I was overridden by concern that the group might break up. It was as if, in counter-transference, I was taking it upon myself to contain (Bion, 1970, p.72) this huge explosive contrast between Love and Death, between the desire that we remain united and, at the same time, that the group be torn apart, because this unity threatened to obliterate us (Hopper, 2003, p.53).

Nevertheless, the first year passed without further dropouts. Toward the end of the year, there were certain imperceptible signs of shifting, both at an individual and at a group level. There was also mention of certain remarkable personal changes that the participants stubbornly refused to associate with our group work. Anna married and appeared to have found some balance; another member, who was on antidepressant medication besides psychotherapy, decided, in agreement with his psychiatrist, to discontinue his medication. Eleni, who in the meantime had become more talkative, went on a diet, lost her first 17 kilograms and had clearly started paying attention to her looks. At the beginning of one of our last sessions before summer break, 47-year-old Stefanos, having taken a book out of my bookcase and while leafing through it, said to me in an almost expressionless voice: "*At some point I might ask you to lend it to me for a few days.*" "*You could take it now*" I said, allowing myself to get carried away, violating the rule of non-involvement. *"No, no,"* he answered as if frightened, and immediately put the book back in its place. Then, three or four of the other members started commenting on the paintings hanging around us on my office walls.

In the autumn, shortly after the summer break, a new member, Annie, 33 years old, joined the group. This made the group "shut down" again like a clam, the sadistic silences returned and it appeared as though none of the first year's gains had been achieved. Annie, a fairly vulnerable girl, brought a false self to the group with which she made an effort to cope with whatever she herself could not bear: silence, other people's problems and particularly the intense emotional reactions of mental pain that might be accompanied by associated references, such as crying.

At the session preceding the one I shall next narrate, Eleni was talking to the group about a serious gynaecological problem that had recently been bothering her. She was restless, because she might have to have an operation and she was terrified of anaesthesia. Annie interrupted her and started comforting her to relieve her stress and protect her, with the calm, smiling air of an expert who is knowledgeable and greatly experienced in such matters. Anna then commented on Annie's behaviour in a manner that sounded overbearing and insulting, as she had done with Eleni in the past. Annie's kind and self-controlled facade then disappeared; she got furious and retaliated angrily and threateningly to Anna, stating that she was not prepared to put up with such behaviour.

The Negation of Fraternal Rivalry

For a long time, the group appeared to systematically negate fraternal rivalry and, at a deeper level, pain and depression, finding an easy refuge in aggression, denigration and violence, at times targeting different group members and at other times the group itself, or me, personally. At other times, when this target was collectively projected within me, my ability to contain as a guardian their own deficiency, despair and anger, was put to the test. However, maybe what was taking place at that particular moment between the two participants with the same name, as had occurred in the past in the instance with Eleni, may have been expressing something more, something even deeper and more frightening, something from the archaic and pre-Oedipal core (Kaës, 2008a) the so-called *fraternal complex*[2] (Kaës, 2008b).

"Yesterday I went to the sea for a swim but there were lots of jellyfish so I lost any desire to go in," says Anna at the next session.

'I'm not afraid of jellyfish anymore," Eleni continues, but then adds: *"On Sunday we went to my mother's sister for lunch. My mother, myself, my aunt and her four children were there."* (That is, seven persons. As many as in the group.) *"As usual, my mother made me want to curl up and die. At some point while serving, I spilt some sauce on the tablecloth. Then my mother said, 'You can't do anything right!' Everyone, including my mother, burst out laughing. I felt humiliated."*

Annie then brought a dream. She was in a hospital and was about to be operated on. She was lying on a stretcher, which was neither in a room nor a ward, but in the corridor. She was to have three operations at the same time: one on her knee, one on the toes of one foot and one on her nasal diaphragm. The surgeon who was to operate on her approached, holding a huge syringe with which he was going to inject her knee. She says: *"Three operations at once?" "Don't be afraid,"* he answers, *"Under anaesthesia you will feel nothing."* Then, totally out of the blue, he gives her a punch and breaks her nose. She is utterly surprised and is covered in blood. *"That's that,"* says the doctor, very calmly. *"To repair the diaphragm we first needed to break the nose."*

In her associations that followed, she mentioned that ever since she was a child, her mother used to beat her. At some point her mother attempted to hit her when she was 14 or 15 years old. Annie grabbed her arm tightly and gave her a powerful punch in the chest. *"That was that,"* she said, *"since then my mother has never raised a hand again."*

A long silence ensued, without carrying any of the sadistic intensity of the past. There we were, seven weak and battered little children, sitting all around, sharing the terror, the immense injustice and despair of finding yourself completely defenceless at the mercy of those you love and who you depend on for everything. I would suddenly catch myself, in my reverie, identifying with their weaker aspects. In other words, I was not in the least envisioning myself in the position of the deceiving, sadistic surgeon where I appeared to be placed in her narrative by the dreamer, as a dream-carrier for the group (Kaës, 2002). On the contrary, I was thinking with genuine sympathy and sorrow of the emptiness of large hospital corridors and the loneliness and insecurity of the patients, abandoned there, on their beds, without their folks, without their own rooms even, homeless, that is, waiting for hours until someone comes to see to them. I wonder, what made me feel this way? It could be that beneath the clearly representational content of the dream, which bore all the characteristics of a violent attack, there was something else transferred secretly to me, amongst the lines of the narrative and the accompanying associations, without my even becoming aware of it. Something possibly marking the passage to the depressed position, thus confirming non-verbally that, after all this laborious work, there was already an opening there for the transition to the possibility for a mental processing of the traumatic.

"I believe that some doctors deserve a good punch in the face," I then said in a low voice, in a tone of faintly plaintive indignation, as if talking to myself. A statement that appeared to sound exculpatory, bringing a relieving laugh to the group.

Conclusion

If the group is traumatogenic, it does not cease, nevertheless, to also be the primary locus where traumas may be re-experienced, mentalized, transformed, worked through and talked about, as Kaës (1993) says.

On the occasion of a comment by Searles regarding the manner in which psychotics tend to mentally "use" the therapeutic teams in psychiatric hospitals, transferring upon them parts of their fragmented Ego that they are unable to differentiate and make whole, "assigning" the therapeutic team to do it for them through transferring identification, Claudio Neri writes the following (Neri, 2011, p.128): "I believe the process described by Searles is not only observed in hospital services, but also in psychoanalytic psychotherapy groups and is not only 'used' by seriously disturbed patients, but by any patient who is able to participate in group analysis."

It is a fact that the traumatic mainly puts psychic envelopes under exhausting pressure, until the breaking point (Ciccone, 2001). By definition, the traumatic is mentally impenetrable. And from this point of view, group envelopes can offer a surface, at the same time internal and external, that at certain critical periods manages to successfully withstand external attacks and contain internal pressures from participants' projections, thus assisting in the symbolization of trauma, in mental processing, in giving meaning, and in a more permanent relief for those who have suffered.

Notes

1 A concept introduced by Didier Anzieu (1985), as a metaphor defining a function and a process. It refers to the containing function of psychic space (individual and group), which has to do with the internalization of the containing object or the containing function of the object.

2 According to Kaës, the fraternal complex includes two conflicting forms. In the first, the archaic form, the subject maintains relations with the brother or sister; the siblings have a part-object psychic status, which is an appendix of the imaginary maternal body or one's own imaginary body. The second form is placed into a triangular rivalry, pre-Oedipal or Oedipal.

References

Anzieu, D., *Le Moi-peau*. Paris: Dunod, 1985.

Bion, W. R., *Experiences in groups*. London: Tavistock, 1961.

Bion, W.R., *Attention and Interpretation*. London: Tavistock, 1970.

Ciccone, A. Enveloppe psychique et fonction contenante: Modèles et pratiques. *Cahiers de psychologie clinique*, 17(2), 2001.

Grappin, J.-J., On bat un groupe. In J.-J. Grappin and J.-J. Poncelet (Eds.), *Groupes et traumatismes*. Toulouse, France: Editions Eres, 2017.

Hopper, E., *Traumatic experience in the unconscious life of groups*. London: Jessica Kingsley, 2003.

Kaës, R., *Crise, rupture et dépassement*. Paris: Dunod, 1979.

Kaës, R., Du Moi-peau aux enveloppes psychiques. Genèse et développement d'un concept. *Le Carnet PSY*, 117, pp. 33–39, 2007.

Kaës, R., *La parole et le lien. Associativité et travail psychique dans les groupes*. Paris: Dunod, 1994.

Kaës, R., *La polyphonie du rêve*. Paris: Dunod, 2002.

Kaës, R., Le complexe fraternel archaïque. *Revue française de psychanalyse*, 72(3), pp. 383–396, 2008.

Kaës, R., *Le complexe fraternel*. Paris: Dunod, 2008.

Kaës, R., *Le groupe et le sujet du groupe. Eléments pour une théorie psychanalytique du groupe*. Paris: Dunod, 1993.

Kaës, R., *Les alliances inconscientes*. Paris: Dunod, 2009.

Neri, C., Le groupe: Manuel de psychanalyse de Groupe. Editions Eres, 2011.

Wood, D., On working with opaque silence in group psychotherapy. *Group Analysis*, 49:3, pp. 233–2, 2016.

Chapter 9

Bequeathing Trauma

Mariagrazia Giachin and Giuliana Marin

Adelina was a young woman sent by a colleague of another town, where she had been studying at the University, to start a course of treatment. She felt ill; a deep fear of death had found its way into her, by forcefully breaking into her consciousness since her early adolescence.

She was a smart and very sensitive woman, carrying the weight of a, as she said, *"intrusive and cumbersome family,"* who she feared it would overtake her life; she feared the long shadows left in herself by the affects, by the family links she still felt bound by, fearing they could constitute intrusive obstacles in the emotional life she was going to build with her partner, considering the state of anxiety into which she was sinking. A single daughter, she had grown up very attached to the idealized mother, while the father, who had continued to represent himself as a victim of an unjustly cruel fate, was a figure constantly devalued by the mother herself. The relationship between the parents was confused, extremely tense and a violent quarrel could arise for whatever reason.

During the therapy, complex and traumatic family histories of both parents emerged. Their own families had suffered the ravages of wars and both Adelina's parents had lost their fathers during World War II. At the beginning of psychotherapy, Adelina spoke as if in a commentary, while she was talking of the events that *"vomited over her,"* overwhelming both her parents and their families. Adelina was trying to distance herself from the anxiety that in other moments seemed to overwhelm her and that the therapist collected and held for her, allowing her to gradually reappropriate it.

Thus, strong painful aspects began to emerge in Adelina's story which had characterized the family history, that seemed not having been elaborated, thus, passing as bequeathed traumas to successive generations.

The Father

Her father was born fatherless, because his mother had become a widow while she was pregnant. The paternal grandmother, a very religious woman, a last-born child of a peasant family, had married a man older than her, that

DOI: 10.4324/9781003269649-13

she didn't love. He had gone to war and had not returned. She had loved her older brother who, when she was a little girl, had gone to the front and there had been no news of him since. In addition to these painful losses, there had been the death of Adelina's father's twin sister, who had died when at age 1; this further mourning had contributed to the development by her paternal grandmother of a symbiotic relationship with the surviving son, supporting him in the idea of being a poor orphan, who had no one other than her and to entrust his fate only to "*divine providence.*" It leads one to think of the grandmother's unexpressed anger for the losses suffered and to the denied hate and anger toward her child: in this way, everything was sacrificed by her on the altar of "divine providence." Trusting in their "divine providence," they decided to emigrate, seeking their fortune abroad; there they were able to find work within a religious community that had welcomed them for about three years. Adelina's father wasn't able to handle this "change." He wasn't able to "place himself" in the environment to find a sense of continuity, and, feeling "lost" in the new continent (the promised land), he had been living a catastrophic experience which undermined his identity.

This event had probably re-activated latent aspects connected to spatial and temporal stability loss, where everything new had been experienced in a traumatic way[1]. He was not able to take advantage of the study opportunities that had been offered to him (he felt his head was exploding when he was studying or thinking deeply about things), as if his head were unconsciously inhabited by persecutory phantoms of the dead twin and of the father who had died while the mother was pregnant. He had been surviving just waiting to return to his home country. While he was abroad, he had begun to correspond with Adelina's mother, who he had met before leaving; this correspondence relationship might have grown over the years, and become strongly idealized.

From Adelina's history, her father figure appears like a man who had suffered because of cumulative trauma and who had been framed as a victim, a bearer of persecutory experiences which had permeated his life since his conception (war, father's loss) and his very early life (twin sister's death). His mother, deeply depressed and "psychically dead," hadn't been able to help her son in elaborating very early traumas, which had overwhelmed both of them. Thus Adelina's paternal grandmother had had to find a way to survive in a war environment which was persecutory, acting and re-acting on a very concrete level. The grandmother's psychic fragility and the symbiotic relationship with her son had hindered the possibility for the mother to be the object of his anger: his hate could have destroyed her, compromising the relationship with the primary object and thus his own survival.

Thus, the mother was strongly idealized and Adelina's father, whom Argentinian psychoanalyst Luis Kancyper[2] would call a "*resentful subject,*" had continued to live (or maybe to survive), keeping a too-close relationship with his mother. It was as if he were imprisoned in an unconscious relationship with her with low intrinsic energy, low libido to invest in the outside world; believing the world owed him a compensation, he could only express anger and resentment.

Idealization and negation, had become defensive mechanisms constitutive of the links. This happened in the couple relationship with Adelina's mother, urged by the traumatic compulsion to repeat that which reproduced what Adelina's grandmother had not been able to elaborate. The post-war escape to another country from their homeland, which had become or was perceived as being a hostile place, the uprooting experience, the emigration to a "promised land," had been experienced by Adelina's father, like a break in the "existence continuity" rather than as a vital opportunity, a rebirth, therefore, making it impossible for him to build empathetic relationships[3].

Adelina had perceived her father's resentful feelings toward the world around him, especially against young people (toward whom he felt great resentment), as well as his annoyance and criticism toward herself, meant that he probably perceived her as among "*those who had more.*"

The Mother

The mother was fatherless as a child, too, but her story was different. Adelina's maternal grandparents had married "*for love*" despite the opposition of the families, but also in this family there was mourning for lost children. The first-born died while still being nursed. After this, Adelina's mother was born, then because of economic hardship, there was an abortion. Indeed, this was the great secret of the grandmother's life, who had only ever said that she "*had lost him*" (she was convinced it would have been a boy), suggesting that the pregnancy ended spontaneously as a miscarriage. Only just before dying had she confessed this secret to Adelina, telling her she had always been her "*first*" granddaughter, her favorite one. Finally, the last daughter was born; one who had never known her father who had died in the war shortly after her birth; just when he had been granted leave from the army to go and see his new daughter, he had been killed by enemy artillery. At the beginning of her life Adelina's mother had therefore had significant emotional space for her parents; she had been worshipped and cared for by them, especially by her father. She still had memories, or rather sensations, linked to her father, and had talked to Adelina about him with pleasure and nostalgia: for example, the way she jumped up and down as her father held her on his shoulders. Adelina's mother was only 2 years old when her father had been called away to the war and only 4 when he was killed.

The maternal grandmother, also overwhelmed by depression due to the loss of her husband, had therefore raised her daughters by cultivating the myth of a father/husband "hero," who had married the girl he loved despite the opposition of families, had not bowed to the dictatorship because "his party was the family" and, in the short time he had lived, he had tried to enjoy what life could offer him. The maternal grandmother should have faced up to her resentment[4]: she had hoped that Adelina's mother, "*the fruit of the love,*" would get the most from life. Adelina's mother was brought up therefore being fed the myth of the dead father, of the family origins, where she placed herself (Adelina's mother had not graduated from high school, because she "*would not lower herself*" to face the reality of having to repeat an exam, remaining always "*with her nose turned up*" thinking it was better to quit school than face the indignity of repeating a failed exam) in the difficult position of accepting reality, because she didn't want to accept she was ordinary. The relationship with Adelina's father had been started as an imagined ideal. When he had emigrated, the two had begun a correspondence in which both probably found relief, and which allowed them to escape their realities. When Adelina's father returned to his country, they had begun dating and shortly after they found jobs, they had got married, despite the opposition of the maternal grandmother (she believed that Adelina's father was not good enough for her daughter and, besides, had a strong antipathy toward his mother). But very soon not-elaborated aspects related to the suffered traumas, to the mourning, to the anger and the denied aggressiveness prevailed over the desire (which had been sustained by the idealization) of changing, of a different way of relating in a new everyday life characterized by living with his mother, with whom her father had always shared everything, also the bed in which another woman had now entered, his wife.

The Couple

Adelina's parents appear to be defensively linked around the denial of the aspects of depression and loss, projecting their own aggressiveness on the partner, who is unable to respond to his/her own idealizations, and to the external world, which is full of threats and dangers, as the experience of the war testifies. The parental couple seems to have formed an unconscious alliance that has the tendency to deny the traumas of loss which have never been elaborated: it deals with what French psychoanalyst Rene Kaës (2009, 2010, Italian translation) defines as a "*denegative pact,*" that is the alliance that, assuming a defensive function, structures the link so as to remove, to deny or to refuse some aspects.

It leads one to think of the extraordinary overlapping of the histories of Adelina's parents: almost two "twin" histories that seem to postpone to a fantasy of "magic resolution" of the traumatic aspects, which are dramatically destined to be repeated. The phantoms of death and loss enact links which are simultaneously deadly and indissoluble, thus creating a "brotherly" couple. Adelina's father seems to repeat with his own wife the parental relationship model following the absence of the father[5]. Without a father, in which he could recognize himself and who could deny him the access to the maternal body, he has only resentful aspects toward the outside world and the mental pain in which he finds himself stuck. This brings him to project to the outside his own threatening inner world.

For Adelina's mother, still tied to her father, her husband-brother seems not to threaten the Oedipal fantasy of being in a couple with her own father. When another man introduces himself in her life, the man of another woman, desired by another woman, she allows herself to be overwhelmed in an extramarital relationship, probably as vital as idealized. When, after many years, it could have turned into a stable relationship, she rejected it. She confided in Adelina, telling her of her "double life" and obliged her to keep quiet about it. In this occasion, she also told her she had an abortion to hide the betrayal.

Thus, Adelina's parental couple seems to be like a couple of rival brothers trying to survive the anguish resulting from a sequence of not-elaborated traumas; anguish from which they are protected by the link which unites them. At the same time, they are rivals and they have no limits in their mutual attacks on each other, in the "resentful" attempt to punish the other for his/her incapability to repair what the war, their mothers or the other ones have not known how to give them, leaving in them a gaping emotional debt. Adelina confusedly feels she does not want to be like her mother and does not want a couple relationship like her parents had, which she perceives as deadly and with no way to escape. Her mother betrays her father, maintaining herself faithful to her own idealized father, while her father appears firmly fixed in his own grudge toward the external world.

Adelina would like a different couple relationship; she thinks about the life she would like to start with her partner, but she is frightened and she feels overpowered by an overwhelming anxiety. Adelina doesn't understand why she has to feel so badly about the prospect of a life that should be so desirable in her eyes. At the beginning of the treatment, Adelina wasn't able to express negative feelings toward her mother, instead attacking her father with anger, for his inconsistency as a father and a husband. She describes her family as two couples mother-child, that cohabited under the same roof: the paternal grandmother and her father; her mother and herself.

Whose is this Anguish?

A catastrophic terrible dream seemed to bring out aspects leading to anguish and generational and transgenerational traumas. Moses was the protagonist of this dream. The colors looked sad and dull and Moses didn't look like the epic hero that Adelina had always imagined. It did not show the joyful life of the prince unaware of his ancestry. The only scenes with children concerned the massacre of Jewish children ordained by the pharaoh, from which Moses had escaped, by being left in a basket in the Nile. In the dream, there was the torment of children of all ages, thrown into the

Nile by the guards to kill them. The dark and bloody scenes were accompanied by the screams and cries of the children who were massacred in this way. In her memory, these scenes were long and distressing.

Her thoughts associated the dream to the heroic Moses, as in the movie "*The Ten Commandments*" with Yul Brynner and Charlton Heston. That movie had been for her like a fairy tale. While associating, the settings became more and more colored and warm and even the most arid landscapes seemed to be the setting of "*One Thousand and One Nights.*" The hero was a young, handsome, brave, strong and self-assured Moses. Beloved as much by the Egyptians as by the Jews, in short, a hero. *"You could only cheer for him and wish he was the prince charming,"* the image of the epic hero. Instead, in the dream he appeared as an ambiguous, ambivalent, problematic, not reassuring but rather frightening Moses. He represented an adult world that promised to be dangerous, unpredictable, full of pitfalls, fears and anxieties about death. It intimated a "*climate of war and death,*" the gruesome and destructive part, the nightmare.

Adelina had associated the sense of death invading her when her mother had confided in her about her abortion, without apparent emotion, binding her to the secret. This revelation was very distressing for her because her mother's secret seemed to authorize her, if she got pregnant, to terminate the pregnancy. In the session, it emerged how long this thought had distressed her and only after a long time had she managed to feel lighter about herself. Adelina's dearly loved maternal grandmother, when on her death bed, had confessed to her to having had an abortion, due to the war-time hardship they had lived through, accompanying this confession with regret, sorrow and pain in remembering. In the session, Adelina had thought about the "*many children deliberately killed by adults, as in war, as in abortions.*"

Adelina had felt a lot of anger in remembering the secret confessed to her by the mother and the anguish that had invaded her. The therapist had taken her to the anguish of the dream, to the "*many children deliberately killed by adults, as in war, as in abortion,*" allowing Adelina to connect to her feelings of guilt toward the baby never born, a possible half-brother, as only she had been rescued, by her mother. She had come to feel angry with her mother while she had reduced the intense resentment she had felt against her father, which, at one time, had led her to fantasize of his death as a liberation. She was getting a feeling of sorrow for him, a less far-away feeling; they had in common the guilty feeling toward their dead baby siblings, which Adelina, with great sorrow, had to face. She felt so sorry for her father, now closer to her, as he had wasted his life to play the role of a victim, a "*bad and resentful victim,*" who hadn't been able to look at anybody with tenderness, a prisoner of himself. The dream had allowed Adelina to have other reflections that could have started new historical constructions with new meanings[6]. As in the dream, both parental families had been forced to leave their homes, having the experience of refugee camps.

Both the parents and the grandmothers had been trapped in the suffering of migration, while the war had left them "*large weights*" and a fragility on which all these traumas had found breeding ground. It seems that the vein of anguish, linked to war extermination and to family sufferings, had intersected with the hero family myth.

The myth of Adelina's maternal grandfather (a man against dictatorship, who put his family at the top of his life, died while he was protecting the escape of famous people), immortalized through the stories of her maternal grandmother, seems to serve both as a group defense against mourning that was denied and not elaborated and is thus inherited by subsequent generations[7] and also a family organization prescriber that is unconsciously transmitted, through a transgenerational way, helping to organize the phantasmatic family life (Nicolò, 2015). The myth requires the creation of a family as a primary goal and value for its members. The fulfilment of this mandate seems hampered by deadly aspects that, denied and not elaborated, pass down through the generations. These unchanged and unchangeable aspects, "suspended" in time, are transmitted from generation to generation, affecting the creation of links in succeeding generations. So the grandfather myth, family continuity supervisor, although on the one hand helps to develop a sense of belonging and security, on the other becomes the ultimate group defense against the deadly separation. In both the dream and in the associations is a common point: the crossing of the Red Sea, the waters opening, the migration to a new land, the new world.

This dream and its associations emerging at this point of the therapy could represent an extremely important moment in the analytic process: the experience and the elaborations that enable the escape from Egypt, crossing the river and moving to the "new land!" A land where Adelina is able to develop her relationships to those nearest and dearest, her couple life, their children, settling down in a land, the continuity, the belonging…

The interpretation linked to Adelina's dream associations had revealed that now she was able to feel closer to "crossing the waters," taking possession of what was promised, but never achieved by both of her parents and their families of origin, both who had remained suspended in a land that was not the one they aspired to. The above had been consolidated over years of therapy and led to another dream that we'll define "the therapy end dream":

> I dreamt I had to be responsible for complicated issues. I had to take a narrow single lane, rather unsuitable for the car although it was a paved road. Although, the cars drove with difficulty I could go on, but I can't remember what type of vehicle I was driving. I got out of a traffic jam caused by badly parked cars, without too much difficulty. I entered a pavilion, with large windows, which hosted different activities: there were people who were selling products, such as those people who call

> you at home and want you to show up to sales presentations in pairs to convince you that you are making a good deal and someone was conducting an investigation, and there were clothes on display. A friend of mine appeared – my husband and I had been witnesses at her marriage; we knew it was going to fail. Both my friend and myself were trying on clothes. We have different tastes, especially with regards to women's skirts.
>
> Her current partner came up to her, so I went to another place to try on other dresses, because I felt they should talk about their things. But I didn't find anything for me. When I returned to the place where they were, my husband arrived. Then he started looking for suitable clothes for me. I knew that with him I could find them.
>
> In the meantime, my maternal grandmother arrived. In fact she, who had been a dressmaker, had sewn my wedding gown. I liked a dress prepared by her. I wanted it colored and short, with a sweetheart neckline. My grandma wanted to make me a flowered shawl, because I shouldn't go and get married with bare shoulders. The dress she had made was just fine, but she wasn't satisfied, so that while I was on honeymoon she took it to pieces, but she wasn't able to put it back together. I had done so much to have a dress that wasn't the usual single-use dress and that's exactly what happened, just like with all the other brides…
>
> In the dream, I sent my grandma a little further away to look for other dresses for me, but she could not find anything suitable. Meanwhile, the couple of friends were still talking about their business. I was continuing to try on clothes with the help of my husband. My friend didn't seem in the spirit to go shopping, she didn't look happy and relaxed. She seemed as if she was still tense over the exchange of words with her partner, that didn't look like a squabble between themselves, but rather something that worried them both. I didn't know if I was able to find the dress for me, but in the dream I had the feeling that I could find it there or somewhere else, with my husband.

Adelina was very moved in telling this dream.

This dream and its associations that emerged at this point of the therapy could mean a very important point of the analytic treatment, where it was ending and Adelina could continue in a "banal" everyday life. Adelina seems aware of the difficulty of her analytic treatment, of the narrow streets where it is hard to pass through (the intergenerational and transgenerational heritance, the experience of her parents). In the family histories, couples had been "separated," broken by traumatic separations, war mournings in which men had died. On the other hand, there are her parents' as a couple, bearers of not-elaborated traumas from which they will not be able to escape and they will never be able to separate from each other. For them, time doesn't pass, there is no desire, no hope and no change: this is the kind of model they can bequeath. Adelina is the *"witness"* to such marriages, which are doomed to failure, and she feels she shares this belief with her partner.

Adelina now can relinquish family myths of the heroic grandfather, a myth which was a refuge but also a prison, and now to go through the strenuous and narrow roads. She feels she is able to do that and to live the change. She has met the past, her beloved grandmother who had sewn her wedding dress and just "as it has to be," she had tried on just once. She was moved by the idea that the such-loved grandmother by whom she had felt so dearly loved, had sewed the wedding dress and an appropriate shawl too; she feels that it could be a good omen trying it on only once, although she had seemed to be adjusting to this only in appearance. It seems that the end of the dream takes her into the banality of life, where couples bickering do exist, but they are not the sign of a broken relationship.

Indeed, many choices will have to be made with him who had meanwhile become her husband, a loving husband attentive to her and to her needs, suitably right for her: a couple in the world.

Conclusions

Adelina, through historical thinking[8], attributing new meanings previously unthinkable[9], could rewrite her and her family's life and redesign new paths for the future. Accompanied by the therapist through the journey to reach her "Promised Land," she had been able to recognize her need to establish relationships based on idealization, denial and aggression.

In therapy, new interpretations of old memories have enabled her to change the perception of both herself and her family, of family mandates she had inherited and the possibility of disengaging from those aspects that didn't belong to her, but by which she had been invaded. Recognizing that the experience of anger she felt within herself against her father was associated with a maternal mandate (Adelina had perceived herself as a weapon her mother used against her father) had led to the fall of idealization, giving rise to a process of separation from her mother that could never happen before, because the mother had always been experienced as an element to be protected. For Adelina, the opportunity to think about her own way of being a woman and mother had opened up. Through empathetic contact with her mother and her father, rediscovered "children," and their mothers, crushed by suffering, it had been possible to accept the loss of her own ideal mother and father.

Grandma's confessions told to Adelina, chosen heir of her memories and those of her mother's love affairs, of which she had been entrusted as confidant, had brought Adelina imagining her life according to the dramatic life of her foremothers' imprint. All female lives, where men had not survived or were still inconsistent, widowed mothers that could not be wives and children died or killed by their mothers. Grandmothers who, like their children, had been frozen within not-elaborated and consequently expelled mournings (Racamier, 1992, 1993, Italian translation) that through crossing multiple generations (Trapanese, Sommantico, 2005) had become an unconscious and cumbersome inheritance to Adelina through an "*intergenerational pact of resistance to mourning*" (Kaës, 2008). Then, through finding a new meaning to memories, Adelina was able to free herself from the deadly immobility of resentment that inhibited the psychical working over of grief.

The past had mortgaged the present and the future through an unconscious transgenerational mandate, suspending her in a sort of timelessness. Adelina, crushed by anxiety, had looked for help, with the confused hope to create "*her own life.*"

Notes

1 Kaës (2013): "…the loss of the narcissistic contract and its breakups expose the subjects and the groups to painful experiences of betrayal, of a lost transmission and to a feeling of being disinherited. It seemed useful to me to think of the issue of the exile, of the nomadism, of the wandering and of the movement as symptoms of a removal of the narcissistic contract. Dislocation must be understood as loss of the psychic place, that of the cultural location, of which Winnicott spoke in 1967, he saw an extension of the notion of the phenomena, of the objects and of the transitional spaces: "*Using the word culture, I think of the tradition that is inherited. I think of something that is the common destiny of humanity, to which individuals and groups can contribute, and from which each of us can get something, if we have a place to put what we find.*"
2 Kancyper re-elaborates Faimberg's theory of unconscious alienating identifications and of the telescoping of generations, introducing the concept of claiming identification, which is realized on the basis of an occupation by the object of the internal world of the subject, which is thus carrying out a program not its own, resulting in "weakening of the ego's functions in the face of repetition, non-choice, imposed, fatal and irreversible."
3 Nicolò and Tambone (2017): "An internal dead core inhabited by the dead mother, the cold mother introjected in her own inner world that feeds a sadistic and frustrating part of herself, that sabotages the patient's development of the ability to feel empathy for himself and for the other."
4 Kancyper (2003): "The resentment expresses the need for revenge by a subject who feels he has been wronged and believes he should call in the debts that have never been settled." "It arises following the risk of loss of the original sense of totality and narcissistic perfection, in which everything flows initially. Reality prevents the preservation of the original mythical condition. Resentment is fuelled by the denial of current reality, by the vain desire to recover a previous reality and by the condensation of spaces in a timeless reality."
5 The acquisition of the second object (the father) is crucial for the formation of the adult identity and to reach a sufficiently mature object relationship Gaddini (1974).
6 Bollas (1995), Kancyper (2003), Spector Person (2005).
7 Kaes (2008) defines this phenomenon as "an intergenerational pact of resistance to mourning."

8 Bollas (1995): "Each person's past is open to continuous acts of historicizing; "it is a creative function of our psychological capacity to see the course of life in continually new ways. When this work is done the history is sufficiently polysemous to energize many unconscious elaboration."

9 de Mijolla-Mellor (1992): "...it will be during this long work of reinterpreting lived experiences and traces of the past ... that the ego will transform its past to make it the origin and cause of its present."

References

Bollas C., Cracking up. The work of Unconscious Experience, Hill & Wang Publishers, New York, 1995.

de Mijolla-Mellor S., Le plaisir de pensée, PUF, Paris, 1992.

Gaddini E., Formazione del padre e scena primaria, in Eugenio Gaddini Scritti, Raffaello Cortina Editore, Milano, 1989.

Kaes R., Le Complexe fraternal, Dunod, Paris, 2008.

Kaës R., Il complesso fraterno, Ed. Borla, Roma, 2009.

Kaës R., Le alleanze inconsce, Ed. Borla, Roma, 2010.

Kaës R., Cosa può la psicoanalisi di fronte al malessere psichico nelle civiltà ipermoderne? Relazione presentata al Seminario "Malessere sociale e malessere individuale: alleati o nemici?", *Firenze*, 2013.

Kancyper L. Il risentimento e il rimorso, Franco Angeli, Milano, 2003.

Nicolò A.M. Miti familiari e legami patologici, in A.M. Nicolò, P. Benghozi, D. Lucarelli (a cura di), Famiglie in trasformazione, Franco Angeli Editore, Roma, 2015.

Nicolò A.M., Tambone S., Differenti difese familiari per fronteggiare un lutto impossibile, 2017.

Racamier P.C., Le Genie des originies, Payot, Paris, 1992.

Racamier P.C., Il genio delle origini, Raffaello Cortina Editore, Milano, 1993.

Spector Person E., Funzione della storia e della narrazione, in Interazioni 2/2005, Franco Angeli, Milano.

Trapanese G., Sommantico M., La costruzione del paradigma generazionale, in A.M. Nicolò, G. Trapanese, (a cura di), Quale psicoanalisi per la famiglia? Franco Angeli, Milano, 2005.

Chapter 10

Rapid Social Change and Individual Identity

Gianluca Biggio

Introduction and Clinical Report

When the personal computer (PC) became part of everyday life, an epochal change began that marked the entry into the digital age. The first electronic computers reproduced the mechanical era paradigm: centralized control and deterministic transmission from the center to the periphery. With personal devices, a new paradigm began; spontaneous peripheral diffusion re-assembled ex-post from the network, i.e. a fluid and perpetually expanding container. The PC has evolved into today's smartphone, a microcomputer that receives and creates multimedia communication and has become an essential part of our daily lives. In parallel, as sociologists have announced, the social-identity paradigm of modern man has changed. From the centralized control of solid and collective values (Riesman, 1950) we have moved on to the liquid identity of changing individual values (Bauman, 2000a). I would like to introduce the theme of the relationship between social changes and individual identity with a short clinical report.

Lorenzo is a man about 21 years old. The father separated from his mother when he was 8 years old and then moved abroad with a new partner. The father was and is an alcohol abuser. Lorenzo comes to the first interview saying that he has stopped drinking for about one year, but this has not improved his life: he feels empty and devoid of projects for the future. After the first interview, the trauma of the father's abandonment, his anger and disorientation, clearly emerge for me. This emergence is so obvious that Lorenzo, after the first meeting, changes his picture on the communication app, WhatsApp, with an indefinable black night spot with a thin white strip of illuminated stone at the bottom. Lorenzo immediately begins to communicate by playing out a role illustrated by the photo itself and constantly requests to change the timing of appointments. However, he manifests his intention to continue with therapy. I realize that it seems easier for him to communicate with the smartphone than by speaking directly.

He speaks through absence and is absent when he is present. He claims to have a "close" relationship with his mother. There are no traces of a

DOI: 10.4324/9781003269649-14

removed representation of his conflicts with his father who fled abroad. A dissociated behavior emerges (alcohol, social groups as an evasion, smartphone, absences for therapy that he himself cannot justify). What strikes me is the difficulty to use the reflection as possibility of relationship. His requests are concrete; he wants a doctor to give him pills to remove the suffering, he throws himself into listening to music with his smartphone and accepts all the consolatory justifications for his abuse of alcohol. Lorenzo brings to his therapy a disorientated pathological fluidity, full of concrete objects that are not affective.

Changes in Psychic Pathology

In a changing social environment, psychic pathology is also changing: processes of identity formation, transmission of transgenerational ghosts, unconscious identifications are all called into play. Syndromes that are lacking in verbalization and symbolization become more and more frequent. These include panic disorders, borderline personality organizations, identity disorders, body-centered pathology (e.g. through self-inflicted injuries), eating disorders, psychosomatic disorders, masked depressions and a range of problems of addiction including drugs, alcohol, gambling etc. (Suman and Brignone 2006). Extending psychoanalytic treatments to these subjects is necessary for the very survival of psychoanalysis, both as a practice and as a scientific theory. The technique of psychoanalysis must adapt to a pathology in which the symbolic expressive component seems lost, in which the repressed gives way to the non-formed, to a pathology in which the psyche-soma is still confused, and thought is not organized or structured, but dissolves as it emerges. This is a major challenge for psychoanalytic psychotherapy, which has long since understood the importance of a flexible setting to try to intercept "fluid" patients.

Social Change Trauma and Identity

We may perhaps say that very rapid social change is a trauma itself, if not supported by institutions. In the passage from the 19th to the 20th century, in the USA and in England, counseling was born (common in all schools) as a support to those generations that moved from the country to the assembly line.

In the passage from the 20th century to the millennium, the theme of social change seems to have progressively captured the attention of psychoanalysis after a period focused on the individual. Often in the 1890s it was said that the unconscious is outside temporal space logic and therefore not subject to socio-cultural changes. Of course those statements could then be refuted by referring to Reich (1933, 1971), Fromm (1941) and other social psychoanalysts, who described the collective psychotic effects expressed by Nazism.

The considerations of Freud himself lead us to consider the links between social and individual psychology:

> "In the psychic life of the individual the other is regularly present as a model, as an object, as a rescuer, as an enemy, and therefore in this broader sense but unquestionably legitimate, individual psychology is at the same time, from the beginning, social psychology."
>
> (1921, pp. 261–62)

Consistent with the era, today psychoanalysis has become globalized; it opened itself to new knowledge and to "not knowing about the new" as attested by Winnicott, Bion, Ogden and Kaes. Some examples of discussion about this new topic: in 2001, IPA panel The impact of new techniques and new 'reality' in Psychoanalysis" edited by Nunez Jasso (2002), the monographic issue of the *Psychoanalytic Review* (2007) and the article of Litowitz in the *Psychoanalytic* (2012) according to which this is still to be explored as technology will change many aspects of psychoanalytic action.

In the book entitled "Le maletre," Kaes (2012) describes the sense of elusive suffering generated by the weakening of the framework of meta-social and meta-psychological guarantors such as public institutions, religious and civil values, the family, the ethics of social coexistence and so on.

This description is in harmony with the thesis of Bauman (2006), on the fragility of identity in the modern age. Internationally renowned writers such as Houellebecq (1998) describe the identity paradoxes of an era that has shifted human aspiration toward immaterial transcendence from art, philosophy and religion to virtual and technological cyberspace.

The sociologist McLuhan (1964) had understood in the 1960s the transition from the mechanical era to the electronic-digital age with consequent reflections on our way of communicating and therefore defining social identity patterns.

Psychoanalysis sometimes sees in the technology of images and cognition the danger of an expropriation of its own dominion: the unconscious. Publications such as "The Man without Unconscious" by the Italian psychoanalyst Recalcati (2013) are, in my opinion, emblematic.

Psychoanalysis also has difficulty with the question of narcissism: there is no doubt that, today, society tends to favor narcissism through the worship of goods and the valorization of the ego through consumption and possession. But it is equally true that as Levin (2000) states, psychoanalysis is the daughter of postmodern civilization and its power of change is based on a narcissistic illusion that initially involves patient and therapist: bringing the external world into the patient's internal world. After 30 years of peace and post-war idealism during which political adhesion to a unified democracy seemed to spread, things have changed and we find ourselves in a more aggressive world, oriented by the market competition rather than by solidarity ethics. We as analysts have to analyze what is happening in order to have a positive voice in this chapter. Today, psychoanalysis must confront predominant social changes at various levels as well as the impact on individual identity. This is discussed next.

1. The socio-economic transformation of globalization between opportunity and loss

Globalization broadens the imaginary but takes away the relational testimony and the identification of the community, bringing a feeling of relative uncertainty. The forms of return to nationalism seen today seem to be a defense against these socially traumatic aspects. Identity seems accessed not through identification with the seductive fragmentary models of media culture, but through a laborious process that requires the reinforcement of the negative capacities of individuals.

2. The loss of solid references to values and institutions in favor of a "liquid" multiplicity (Bauman 2000b)

A certain level of social trauma is structurally connected to the loss of the "solid" references of the 20th century. The idea is that technology can be a sort of new meta-social guarantor. (Kaës, 2015) But technology developed without social ethics can be a partial and threatening guarantor because it is not institutionalized.

3. Globalized individuality in identity models transmitted perceptually by digital mass media

The current mass media are perceptually pervasive; consider the neuronal formatting of the relationship with the computer, the touch screen, video games in young people and perceptual marketing. Virtual testimony (tutorial) does not compensate for relational learning. Young people entrusted in the hands of the media by couples of "busy" parents become self-centered and transform into "angry" patients because of the implicit abandonment (Bolognini, 2018). This is the mood of many psychotherapies of modern young adults.

4. The risks and sufferings generated by a model of individual performance in consumption and at the workplace

If inner solidity is transposed to the possession of powerful machines and self-esteem is transferred to the possession of designer objects, the greedy attitude of teenagers is not surprising. Nor is the obsession with work performance that allows you to obtain these assets. Psychoanalysis in an unconventional way teaches a reflective and relative use of possession.

5. Models for understanding global behaviors (Big Data) that exclude the unconscious

We see a shift in the understanding of social behavior, for example the famous social representations of Moscovici (2000), from a paradigm of cultural value to an operative quantity, according to the most advanced marketing schemes. The model of representation of men is, as Benasayag and Schmit (2006) affirms, that of the computer—an operative model that avoids deepening the unconscious aspects of social behavior.

Conclusions

Ferdinand Tönnies (2008), a German sociologist in the work *Gemeinschaft und Gesellschaft* (1891–1905), identifies two different forms of social organization: the community (*Gemeinschaft*) and society (*Gesellschaft*). While the community form, based on the feeling of belonging, predominates in the pre-industrial age, the society, based on rationality and exchange predominates in the industrial age. The mass media community is a sum of individuals connected to the media in which the feeling of individuality and loneliness prevails. Benasayag and Schmit (2006) address the issue of the difficult construction of identity in the "era of the sad passions" characterized by a sense of loss of belonging to themselves in the society of compulsive desire and the image of the *homme augmenté* (augmented man).

In "Civilization and its Discontents," Freud (1927) spoke of the wonders of the mechanical age and of the omnipotence through the fantasy of the "prosthetic God" (Egidi Morpurgo, 2013). The mechanical age has given wellbeing by subtracting fatigue from humans and animals. Freud said that the price to pay for civilization was the renunciation of a certain amount of immediate satisfaction in exchange for "a handful of security." What does the citizen of the digital age—paradoxically the age of immediate satisfaction—renounce? What is the price to be paid in exchange for the possibility of communicating in real time in the global village, with the possibility of endlessly moving productions of the external and inner world?

I believe that today, as in the past, Freud would try to delve into the salient themes of the era by bringing an innovative contribution, because of the structure of psychoanalysis, based on the scientific reflection on the relationship between men and something that cannot be scientifically dominated, such as the unconscious. Psychoanalysis is at the same time one of the few paradigms that can bring back to the spirit of the *Gemeinschaft* (community), perhaps through a virtuous use of technology.

References

Bauman, Z., Liquid Modernity. Polity, Cambridge, 2000a.

Bauman, Z., Liquid Times: Living in an Age of Uncertainty. Polity, Cambridge, 2000b.

Bauman, Z., Liquid Fear. Polity Press, Cambridge, 2006.

Benasayag, M., Schmit, G., Les Passions Tristes. Souffrance Psychique Et Crise Sociale. Decouverte, Paris, 2006.

Bolognini, S., Conference SIEFPP "The new forms of malaise and psychotherapy". Bologna, 2018.

Centro di Psicoanalisi Romano, Convegno "Winnicott e la psicoanalisi del futuro". Roma, 30-31 gennaio, 2016.

Egidi Morpurgo, V., "Da Prometeo al Big Brother" in Marzi (a cura di), Psicoanalisi, identità e internet. Esplorazioni nel cyberspace. Franco Angeli, Milano, 2013.

Freud, S., Group Psychology and the Analysis of the Ego. The Standard Edition of the Complete Psychological Works of Sigmund Freud, Volume XVIII, 1920–1922, 1921. The Hogarth Press: The Institute of Psycho-Analysis, London, 1961.

Freud, S., The Uneasiness in Culture. The Standard Edition of the Complete Psychological Works of Sigmund Freud, Volume XXI, 1927–1931, 1927. The Hogarth Press: The Institute of Psycho-Analysis, London, 1961.

Fromm, E., (1941), Fuga dalla libertà. Edizioni di Comunità, Milano, 1963.

Houellebecq, M., Les Particules élémentaires (The Elementary Particles). Flammarion, Paris, 1998.

Kaës, R., L'extension de la psychanalyse. Pour une métapsychologie de troisième type. Dunod, Paris, 2015.

Kaës, R., Le maletre. Dunod, Paris, 2012.

Levin, C., "L'avenir d'une a-civilization: la psychanalyse comme virtualitè du corps primitif" (The future of an a-civilization: psychoanalysis as a virtuality of the primitive body "in The future becomes disillusioned) in L'avenir s'une déesillusion. Press Universitare de France, Paris, 2000.

Litowitz, E., "Psychoanalysis and the Internet: Postscript". Journal Psychoanalytic Inquiry Vol. 32, No. 5, Psychoanalysis and Cyberspace, 2012.

Marzi (a cura di), Psicoanalisi, identità e internet. Esplorazioni nel cyberspace. Franco Angeli, Milano, 2013.

McLuhan, M., Understanding Media: The Extensions of Man; 1st ed. McGraw Hill, NY, 1964.

Moscovici, S., Social Representations. Cambridge, Polity Press, 2000.

Nuñez Jasso, E., "El impacto de nuevas tecnicas y nuevas "realidades" en psicoanalisis (The impact of new technologies and new realities in psychoanalysis)". International Journal of Psychoanalysis, 83, pp. 926–30, 2002.

Psychoanalytic Review, Special Issue on the Internet, Vol. 94, No. 1, February 2007.

Recalcati, M., L'uomo senza inconscio (The man without the unconscious). Raffaello Cortina, Milano, 2013.

Reich, W. (1933), Psicologia di massa del fascismo. Trad. it Einaudi, Torino, 1971.

Riesman, D. (1950) La folla solitaria. Trad. it. Il Mulino. Bologna, 2009.

Suman, A., Brignone, A., "Transference, Countertransference, Society and Culture: Before and During The First Encounter". BJP British Journal of Psychotherapy, November, 2006.

Tönnies, F., Soziologische Schriften 1891–1905 (Sociological writings). Rolf Fechner, Profil-Verlag, München/Wien, 2008.

Part IV

Migration and the Paths of Trauma

Chapter 11

Telemachus' Predicament

Trauma and Emotional Rupture in the Relationship between Immigrants and Their Left Behind Children

Lida Anagnostaki and Alexandra Zaharia

Parent-child Separation as a Feature of the Migratory Challenge

Mexican migrant families forcefully divided at the American borders recently made headlines around the world (Holpuch, 2018; Shear, Goodnough, & Haberman, 2018), but, sadly, this is only the tip of the iceberg. Young children's separation from their parents, who emigrate to pursuit a better future in faraway lands, is a common condition in the migratory challenge (Dreby, 2010; Graham, & Jordan, 2011).

Paradoxically, this condition has been largely overlooked in the psychoanalytic literature, although immigration has been a central experience in the psychoanalytic field. Many analysts, Freud himself included, have emigrated from their native countries. This experience has led many of them to explore the complexity of the migratory process from both a theoretical and a clinical angle (Rustin, 2013), and significant texts have been written on the subject (see León and Rebeca Grinberg's book "Psychoanalytic Perspectives on Migration and Exile" [1989], or the most recent texts by Vamik D. Volkan [1999; 2017], and Salman Akhtar [1999; 2011], which thoroughly investigate the psychic vicissitudes and impact [both negative and positive] of migration on the migrating person).

The emotions, however, the thoughts and needs of the migrants' children who are left behind in the country of origin under the care of relatives (usually the grandparents, more rarely an aunt or uncle) have been almost ignored by psychodynamic theorists and researchers. Although in other human sciences, disciplines who typically employ quantitative (and in that sense, more 'distant') research approaches the struggles of the immature offspring of economic migrants have received attention (Antman, 2012; Wen, & Lin, 2011), this has not been the case within the psychoanalytic literature, which normally paves the way to a deeper understanding of the complexities and challenges of the human condition.

In our review, we only found two relevant references. A short reference to this condition of separation is found in the book of Grinberg and

DOI: 10.4324/9781003269649-16

Grinberg (1989). Drawing clinical material from the therapy of young Javier, a boy whose parents emigrated leaving him behind, the Grinbergs argue that the "children who do not emigrate together with their parents" form a "separate category" for whom "the migratory experience ends in catastrophe" (pg. 70) and who may develop symptoms that are clearly connected to their predicament. The second reference can be found in Elaine Arnold's work (2006; 2011), which draws on attachment theory and focuses on African Caribbean adolescent women who, after a long period of separation, immigrated to United Kingdom to rejoin their families. According to her, the separation can lead to long-term traumatic consequences, especially if, as is the case with the women in her sample, one has also to deal with the stress of one's own immigration.

Although these references point to a direction of studying the young children's separation from their parents who emigrate within a psychoanalytic perspective, we believe that a more detailed study into those parent-child relationships can help us get a comprehensive understanding of the challenges and adversities that the, unfortunately not few, 'left behind' children have to endure.

The Myth of Telemachus

Ulysses' *nostos* (homecoming), which took him 10 eventful years, is often used as a metaphor for immigration. However, when narrating the adventures of this clever and versatile king, little emphasis is generally given to the fact that brave Ulysses was the father of young Telemachus, who hadn't seen him since his infancy, and is described by Homer as sitting for hours on the shore waiting for his father's ship to appear. According to the myth, Ullyses left young Telemachus unwillingly; in fact, he only agreed to follow the other Greek kings to Troy when his son's life was threatened. Still, Telemachus experienced the parental absence as a trauma that left him perplexed and empty, not knowing *what* or even *if* something connects him to his father. He protests that he does not know who "sowed" him, although other people narrate to him his father's deeds (*The Odyssey*, Rhapsody A: 215–216).

In the present study, we interviewed adults who were left behind as children when their parents emigrated, trying to delineate the emotional consequences of parental migration. We focused on the distance — not the physical, which is imposed by the very condition of migration — but the emotional distance that seems to be created when the parents 'leave their children behind.' During the interviews, we often felt that these 'left behind' children were just like modern Telamachuses, who kept on waiting for their parents to return after years of separation, wondering about the parents who left them. As Recalcati (2015) claims, when the place of the parent is void, it is difficult for the children to feel they are 'real' children:

"whose children? whose parent and whose adult?" (pg. 85). This is one of the key questions that runs through the discussion of the findings.

Immigration, Relational and Collective Trauma

Immigration is generally understood as "a forced or a voluntary move through which the individual changes his habitat" (Varchenvker, 2013, pg. 9). Economic immigrants' resettlement is considered "voluntary," in the sense that they are not forced or expelled by a tyrannical regime but choose to leave because of economic hardship in their country of origin. However, it is utterly logical to assume that it was not just mythical Ulysses that left his young child unwillingly. The majority of the parents who emigrate due to financial necessity also leave their children behind against their will. Still, it seems that the parental absence, whether underwent in a palace in Ithaca, or in a small house in an impoverished village, is nevertheless experienced as a major deprivation. If a parent emigrates, children have no choice but to follow the path chosen for them.

We think that in this context Brearley's (2013) approach of bringing together the concept of trauma as a psychological event affecting the individual, and the concept of collective trauma that affects societies and groups is useful. Trauma in the modern psychoanalytic literature is deemed as a complex and multifaceted phenomenon (Kaplan, 2006; Rosnik, 2013). Besides the elaboration on the psycho-economic model of trauma, initially developed by Freud (1920; 1926), psychodynamic theorists have explored trauma in object relations, emphasizing the traumatogenic quality of bad object relationships, or the break of them (Bohleber, 2007), what is also called relational trauma (Mucci, 2013). In addition, they have thoroughly studied the psychological reactions to traumatic events that affect an entire society, that is, collective or social trauma (Hirschberger, 2018).

It seems that in the case of economic migration and the 'left behind' children that all these parameters of trauma are at play. Parents leave their native country and their offspring behind because of poverty, which is conceptualized as a special type of collective trauma characterized by persistent and never-ending exposure of people living in poverty to significant adversities (Shamani, 2018). Their leaving, however, possibly results to the traumatization of their children, who are left alone, feeling mistreated by the very people whose protection and care is mostly needed (Bohleber, 2007). We propose that this is a case where collective trauma, that is "the blow to the basic tissues of social life that damages the bonds attaching people together" (Erikson, 1976, pg. 154), brings about individual trauma, that is "a blow to the psyche that breaks through one's defences so suddenly and with such brutal force that one cannot react to it effectively" (Erikson, 1976, pg. 153). In this study we focused on the effects of this condition on the parent-child relationship, exploring whether it results in a "failure of belief in the protection afforded by good objects" (Garland, 1998), leaving a profound scar on the children left behind.

The case of Greece

Modern Greece is a country with significant emigration experience. In its course, there have been three mass economic migration waves during which more than 1,750,000 Greeks have migrated to foreign countries (Kotzamanis, & Mihos, 2005; Lazaretou, 2016). This number is to be compared to the total population of Greece that today mounts merely to 10,750,000 people[1]. Economic migration, "motherland's inability to feed her children," is considered traumatic and regarded as social drainage (Lazaretou, 2016).

By far, the most numerous economic immigration wave took place in the middle of the 20th century as a result of the destruction and the poverty incurred during World War II and the civil war that followed. A large number of Greek men and women moved to more industrialized countries to the European North. It is estimated that between 1960 and 1963, more than 500,000 Greeks worked in West Germany as 'guest-workers' (Gallant, 2016). Their plan was to save their earnings and return to Greece shortly, but in most cases, immigration proved to be a long-term solution.

The second immigration wave is the focus of the present study. The research explored the impact of parental immigration on young children who in 1960s and 1970s were left behind in Greece, to live with relatives, while their parents lived and worked abroad, and these children's (now adults') understanding and meaning making, in retrospect, of this experience. Their story, which seems not to have been thoroughly explored before, poses some very poignant questions that are strangely timely, or, one can say timeless, just as the myth of the 'left behind' Telemachus.

Methodology

Research rationale and design

The research aspired to present a valid combination of psychoanalytic thinking and robust qualitative design, as we believe that complementing psychoanalytic insights with evidence from other research methods, with respect to each discipline's major tenets, can add complexity to the scientific investigation, and also strengthen the exchange between psychoanalysis and other disciplines that contribute to scientific knowledge today (Bernardi, 2015).

Lately, a number of researchers have been looking for research methodologies that are able to retain the specificity and complexity of the human experience, aiming at the discovery and increased understanding of the multifaceted human world (Midgley, 2004). The Interpretative Phenomenological Analysis (IPA), the qualitative research method we employed in this study, follows this paradigm (Smith, Flowers, P., & Larkin, 2009). It is deemed especially relevant when faced by a relatively unexplored area and the focus of the research is to illuminate the meanings which people employ to make sense of their life experiences (Midgley, 2004). It includes a detailed analysis of a small number of cases, grounded in the data itself, involving, though, constant interplay between observation and interpretation stemming from a dialogue with the researcher's theoretical background.

According to Midgley's (2004) figure of the three concentric circles depicting the range of psychotherapeutic research, the present research's topic can be described as a topic in the broadly-focused area of psychotherapeutic research. In this area are included explorations of topics that are "highly relevant to the psychotherapeutic profession, but are not directly focused on clinical work, such as research looking at children's experiences of growing up with a depressed parent or being removed from their families and placed in care."

Participants

Fourteen people, five men and nine women, aged between 28 and 56 years, participated in the study. The participants were recruited through the interviewers' personal and social networks and through snowballing. In order to recruit a homogenous sample, as recommended for IPA (Smith et al., 2009), the following inclusion criterion was used: when participants were younger than 10 years of age, both their parents have moved to a foreign country as economic immigrants, while the participants stayed in Greece with relatives for a period of at least 1 year. All participants provided informed consent and confidentiality issues were discussed at the beginning and the end of each interview. Participant demographics are detailed in Table 11.1 (to safeguard participants' anonymity, pseudonyms are used).

Data Collection and Analysis

Phenomenological accounts were elicited through semi-structured interviews that were conducted by the first author. She also kept a research diary where she noted her thoughts and transference/countertransference reactions after each interview. The interview schedule was designed in such a way to obtain a detailed and in-depth account of the participants' experience. Examples of interview questions are shown in Table 11.2. The first part consisted of questions about the participants' childhood experiences, focusing on the experience of separation, while in the second part, questions about the meaning of those recounted experiences with regard to their

Table 11.1 Participants' demographics

Name	*Gender*	*Age*	*Age and duration of separation*	*Family status*
1. Flora	F	43	4–7 years of age	Married, 2 children
2. Eleni	F	43	6 months–1 year and 3–5 years	Single
3. Makis	M	47	2 months–1 year and 2–5 years	Single
4. Mina	F	56	6–7 years	Single, 1 child
5. Zeta	F	39	8 months–17 years	Single
6. Melina	F	39	0–10 years	Married, 3 children
7. Dorothea	F	56	2–7 years	Married, 1 child
8. Theano	F	44	2.5–4.5 years	Married, 3 children
9. Aliki	F	51	1 month–12 years	Married, 3 children
10. Doros	M	56	6–12 years	Married, 2 children
11. Elpida	F	34	9–13 years	Single
12. Tassos	M	53	7–11 years	Married, 2 children
13. Harris	M	28	2–8 years	Single
14. Stavros	M	50	3–5, 5 years and 7–8 years	Married, 1child

current lives were asked. As recommended for IPA, the interview schedule was not employed prescriptively, but instead adapted and adjusted with each interview. All interviews were audio-recorded.

The interview recordings were transcribed verbatim by the second author, together with the nuanced aspects of the participants' accounts. The transcripts were systematically read and analyzed in line with Smith et al.'s (2009) guidance, first one by one, and the emerging themes related to the research questions were noted. Once each individual transcript was analyzed, the patterns across interviews were established and the themes were integrated. The analysis was conducted by the first author and discussed with the second author as it proceeded. The developing themes

Table 11.2 Example of interview questions

1. Tell me a little bit about yourself.
2. How would you describe your childhood?
3. How would you describe the relationship with your parents?
4. What do you remember from the period that your parents left?
5. How did you feel then?
6. What were your thoughts then?
7. How do you feel now about them leaving?
8. What are your thoughts now about them leaving?
9. How would you describe the relationship with your parents now?
10. Do you think that their leaving has affected your life?

were reviewed together. The participation of the second author offered triangulation, as a way of ensuring the credibility of the findings (Midgley, 2006). Other quality issues were addressed by utilizing the guidelines described by Smith (2011).

IPA emphasizes that access to the participants' experiences depends on the researcher's own conceptions and, in fact, these are required to make sense of the other's personal world (Smith, & Eatough, 2007). Both researchers are trained psychoanalytic psychotherapists; we argue that both our theoretical background, that stresses the importance of subjective experience, and our clinical experience, that focuses on the monitoring of transferential and countertransferential feelings and on interpretative activity, were essential tools for the implementation of such analysis. These assets proved to be extremely helpful, on the one hand for the carrying out of the interviews (view for instance, the necessary adaptation of the questions based on the flow of each interview filtered by the countertransference of the interviewer), and on the other, for the analysis of the transcripts and the establishment of emerging themes that corresponded consistently to the participants' experience and to more abstract, theoretical formulations.

Results

The wealth of the human experience presented to us through the narratives was vast and admittedly the categorization of the material was challenging, as any classification has *de facto* an artificial quality. However, we believe that thanks to IPA's commitment in exploring both the convergences and divergences between the participants' narratives, the results manage to reflect the complexity of the 'left behind' children's experience.

As Table 11.3 shows, the analysis yielded an overarching theme, *Trauma of being left behind*, that was prominent in the accounts of all participants and encompassed all superordinate themes. The analysis of the participants' accounts yielded four further superordinate themes: *Intense emotions, Effects on parent-child relationship, Defences*, and *Psychopathology*, which were further analyzed in non-mutually exclusive subordinate themes (for a detailed discussion see Anagnostaki, & Zaharia, 2020).

As mentioned, this chapter focuses on the relationship between immigrant parents and their 'left behind' children, as it was then and as it is now so many years later. Despite the abundance of material, we will have to limit ourselves to presenting the themes that fall strictly into this focal field. Therefore, the superordinate theme *Effects on parent-child relationship* and the subordinate themes that it encompasses will be presented. The numbers in parentheses show the number of participants who offered material adhering to each theme.

Table 11.3 IPA results: overarching theme, superordinate and subordinate themes

Trauma of being left behind			
Intense emotions	*Effects on parent-child relationship*	*Defences*	*Psychopathology*
Anger/feeling of injustice	Rupture of the relationship in childhood	Replacement of parental figures	During separation
Pain/sorrow	Difficulties in rapprochement	Rationalization	In later life
Abandonment	Emotional distance in adulthood	Reparation through their own children	
Perplexity	(Pseudo)independence		
Fear/insecurity		Emotional isolation	

Effects on parent-child relationship

The participants spent a large part of their childhood 1,000 kilometers away from their parents, at a period when transportation was unaffordable for the meager finances of the immigrant families and communication very difficult. Usually, the only available means of communication was postal mail. Telephone communication was almost impossible; in most cases there was only one telephone in the whole village. Eleni, for instance, remembers that during the two years she stayed away from her parents, she only spoke to them on the phone twice.

However, what primarily emerged from the interviews is not the physical distance between the participants and their parents, but the experienced emotional distance between them, in childhood, and later in life. In the eyes of the children, the parents' absence was interpreted as indifference and lead to rupture in parent-child relationship. Furthermore, the reunion with their parents, when they returned from abroad, also caused distress. On the other hand, five participants talked highly of the independence they gained thanks to the early and prolonged separation from their parents. It is noteworthy, however, that their descriptions are reminiscent of the behaviour of the insecure-avoidant children (Ainsworth, Blehar, Waters, & Wall, 1978), therefore possibly pointing toward pseudo-independence and not toward mature autonomy. The four subordinate themes that were identified are presented in detail below. The analysis is supported by verbatim interview extracts from the research participants, following IPA's guidelines (Smith et al., 2009). The concealers in brackets indicate material that has been omitted.

Subordinate theme–Rupture in the relationship in childhood (10):

> "There was no relationship. Once there is distance, there is no relationship, it is pretty obvious there was no relationship. There was some kind

of communication, good or bad, that makes no difference […], but this was no relationship." Zeta

"…I don't remember the word "mom" or that sort of words. I did not even have an image of them […] Some people would come from Germany to the village, and my mother would send chocolates; once she sent me a coat, it was a black one, a nice one, but ok, it meant nothing to me. The chocolates came. We ate them. End of story. Who sent them? Mom. What is mom? I did not know. Mom… nothing, she was a chocolate I got and ate." Dorothea

"… I felt that I love my mom at a very old age. You know what I mean when I say to love her… I thought I loved her, because she was my mom, because 'that's the way it should be: we love our mom, our dad.' But to feel it… I felt it at a very old age." Alice

"No, it wasn't… it didn't exist… that is, we did not have this kind of contact […]. I think they completely gave us away to grandpa and grandma, and unfortunately, for us and for them, our relationship was almost non-existent. I don't have many memories from my parents when I was little. I do have a memory, my first memory, probably when I was at first grade, when my mom was waiting for me downstairs, and I didn't recognize her." Melina

In the case of two participants, the rupture they experienced in the relationship with their parents led them to openly question whether they were actually loved by their parents.

"Ok, so many years have passed, right? But sometimes I wonder whether I had received this kind of love I am showing my daughter now." Stavros

Subordinate theme–Difficulties in rapprochement (4):

"When my mother came back, that was the difficult part. For starters, she returned with my sister… I had not met her before… Another child came… I saw her with this child, and I thought of them as enemies. They were enemies that entered the house. That was true. Enemies. In the house. […] The next day I left, I went to sleep with my grandma and she came to get me, I told her, no, I don't want you, you are not my mother, go away, you stink, and I would tell her that she is a gypsy woman. Although she put on cologne, she bathed with shampoo and soap, etc., aaaaah…, to me her smell was that of a stranger's, and I would tell her go away, you stink, you are a gypsy woman, I don't want you." Dorothea

"What I can tell you is that basically at five I was reunited with my parents […]. My most intense memory… I was embarrassed. That is, we were not used to each other, I knew they were my parents and that was supposed to mean something, but I did not feel comfortable around them." Makis

Subordinate theme–Emotional distance in adulthood (5):

"I think that if, after that, after they had come back, they had tried to get to know me, and if I had seen a different kind of effort on their part, maybe our relationship would have been better. But I've always had this feeling, I always felt lonely inside my family, and with my parents, always something [...] And today that is our relationship like that, for me it's not okay. I mean there is nothing specific I say 'this should be different.' In order for our relationship to be different... that would take three different persons. I'm totally okay. I think my parents are suffering. It costs them. It costs them. I can tell you that because my mother sometimes calls me and she tells me: 'Ahh, other people talk to their parents every day.' 'And what do they talk about every day?', 'How come they find something to talk about and we don't?" Eleni

"I mean, the biggest void I still have in my life is this. That I do not have... I know that what I am most jealous of, is that I wish I had a relationship, like the one normal people have with mom, and dad of course, but much more with my mom. But this cannot happen, there is nothing we can do..." Melina

"Listen, I will explain to you how I interpret it, how I see it. When parents give birth to children, and they give them away, they leave them, and they see their children all grown up, [...] the gaps that this relationship has, the gaps essentially have to do with this one thing, that there is no knowledge, that basically you, as a mother, you don't know your child." Makis

Subordinate theme–(Pseudo)independence (5):

"My parents, I can tell you that even now, I do not know them. I don't know them as persons. That is, I now know what they are like, as characters etc., but I have never felt this kind of bonding, mother-father-child. Only in theory, and as a biological fact. And I don't mind. I know what kind of people they are, that they tried for the best for me and my siblings and for everything, but I just didn't have this kind of bonding. [...] I have no dependency. For me ... maybe that would be a negative thing for somebody else. That would scar him for life, make him have phobias, that kind of things. To me, it was exactly the opposite. A sense of freedom, a sense of taking decisions on my own. After all there was a time, when I was 16, 17, even though my family came here, I took the decision and went away, on my own, at this young age. And this is a great proof that I do not have any ties that restrict me." Tassos "[talking about how her parents' leaving affected her] ...it does that to you, it does, but it makes you find faith... find a way to survive. And I found my way. I might have been sad, but I found the way. Independence." Elpida

Discussion

It is impossible to speak of traumatic events in an absolute way, without considering the unique characteristics of the internal world and the sensitivity of each subject. Nevertheless, following Mucci (2013), we argue that the individual threshold should not prevent us from exploring trauma as a real event that may occur at a collective level and have significant impact on the individual level. Making use of psychoanalytic tools, we believe it is possible to highlight the movement from collective to individual.

Poverty has been discussed as a cumulative trauma that affects self-identity and the quality of object relationships: often the parents in the families that live in poverty are not in the position to cater for their children's biological and emotional needs, and it sometimes seems that their main, or maybe sole, objective is to escape from this predicament, leaving all other considerations aside (Yang, 2014). That was precisely the reason why the parents of the participants in this study emigrated. They fled Greece striving to build a better life for themselves and their children. In turn though, the early and prolonged parent-child separation resulted in the rupture of the fundamental link of trust and hope between self and other. This constituted a traumatic event for their young offspring and led to the creation of an unbridgeable gap.

The issue of parental alienation emerged in the majority of the interviews. Ten participants talked about the lack of closeness and intimacy we usually take for granted in the parent-child relationship. They seemed to question the very nature of their relationship with their parents during their childhood (*"There was no relationship,"* Zeta); they wondered whether they were loved by them (*"I wonder whether I had received this kind of love,"* Stavros), or whether they themselves loved them (*"I felt that I love my mom at a very old age,"* Alice). It seemed that, just like young Telemachus, they were trying to figure out what those people were to them, and how/if they were connected: *"What is mom? I did not know. Mom... nothing,"* concluded Dorothea.

Ulysses' *nostos*, the central theme of the Odyssey, is supplemented by Telemachus' search for his father. His search ends favourably with the acceptance of the unavoidable reality of separation, and the recognition that he is the heir of his father's and mother's crossed destinies. But this is the good scenario. The working through of the "break of the I/thou relationship that constitutes the traumatic effect" (Laub, & Auerhahn, 1989) is not a simple task. The participants in our study experienced separation from and the long absence of their parents in their infancy and early childhood. According to Gurevich (2008), prolonged absence is shocking and frightening. The self, in order to compensate for the pain caused by absence and to survive, causes an inner absence by disconnecting parts of himself. The self may also resort to other defences, such as the denial of dependency needs, emotional isolation, rationalization, omnipotence; defences that hinder the process of mourning and symbolization, and therefore the working through of experience. Recalcati in his book "The Complex of Telemachus" (2015) wonders how we can give hope to a crumpled Telemachus. We think that in case of the participants in our study, the answer relates to their ability to work through the trauma of 'being left behind.'

This working through, as well as the level of traumatization, depends on several factors, including the length of the absence, the age when separation occurred and the presence or absence of other relations which serve a reparatory function (Mucci, 2013). When their parents went away, the majority of the participants were taken care of by their grandparents (or in one case by an aunt) who have taken the role of the primary carer: *"they completely gave us away to grandpa and grandma,"* Melina reported. However, the replacement of the absent parent by another person did not mean that the absence of parents was not experienced as traumatic. On the contrary, it seems that the children desperately held on to this idea of the parent who abandoned them. As Greenberg and Mitchell (1983) argue, often the emptier the exchange with the parent, the greater is the child's devotion to the promising yet depriving features of this relationship, perhaps resulting to *"the biggest void"* Melina talks about.

Participants in the research also talked about the difficulties of reconnecting with their parents when they were reunited after the long-term separation. In the Odyssey, the episode of recognition of Ulysses by his son Telemachus is indeed powerful. The father, after 10 years of absence, is unrecognizable. He is a stranger to his son. The recognition, after so many years of absence cannot be based on a common past or common memories. Of course, in the myth the problem is uncomplicatedly solved, thanks to the divine intervention of Athena. In the reality, of our participants' lives the rapprochement caused distress that was not easily overcome. The participants in our study faced a *"stranger"* who *"stank"* (in Dorothea's words), who made them feel "*embarrassed*" and *"uncomfortable"* (according to Makis), and *"that was the difficult part,"* as Dorothea narrates.

Reconnection was further complicated if new family members, that is young siblings, arrived together with the parents (Suarez-Orosco, Todorova, & Louie, 2002). In these cases, an additional factor that hindered rapprochement was the painful recognition that the parental couple functioned and "produced" children while away from them. As Dorothea movingly puts it: *"I saw her [i.e. her mother] with this child, and I thought of them as enemies. They were enemies that entered the house."*

In some cases, early parental separation caused a permanent rift in the parent-child relationship. Five participants described the emotional distance from their parents they experience as adults. Unsurprisingly, those are the participants who had spent most of their childhood away from their parents. In their narratives, the perplexity and unfamiliarity concerning parent-children relationships seems poignant: *"What do they talk about every day?"* asks Eleni when her mother tells her that people talk to their parents every day. It seems that these children lack the feeling of 'belonging together' with their parents: there are *"gaps,"* says Makis about which *"there is nothing we can do,"* explains Melina. According to Mucci (2013), a traumatized person "manifests a painful state of concurrent awareness of a depleted self" (pg. 73), a statement we believe applies to the narratives of these participants.

Conversely, five participants described the positive aspect of early separation from their parents, arguing that they have become independent *"with no ties to restrict [them],"* as Tassos characteristically says. We propose that this dramatic renunciation of emotional ties to the parents (*"I found the way. Independence,"* as Elpida says) might be an attempt to mask the distress caused by the unresponsiveness of the object, as is the case with the insecure-avoidant children (Ainsworth et al., 1978). It has been shown that in some cases, for instance when parents are emotionally unavailable due to some kind of mental disorder, the adoption of an avoidant attachment style is perhaps more functional than the adoption of an attachment style that presupposes the emotional availability of the parent (Näslund, Persson-Blennow, McNeil, Kaij, & Malmquist-Larsson, 1984). However, although adaptive, it is still a coping mechanism (Bowlby, 1969) which compromises healthy, across-the-board development. Mature independence and separation presuppose a well-established feeling of belonging and relatedness, which these children seem not to have adequately conquered (*"I have never felt this kind of bonding, mother-father-child,"* admits Tassos). Yet, Ulysses has to return home and reconnect with Telemachus, in order for Telemachus to become truly independent, to be the "proper heir to the throne" (Recalcati, 2015).

Children separated from their parents due to migration has been, and sadly continues to be, part of the migration challenge. In that sense, the narratives of the participants in our study are not unique. However, we hope that through the interpretative analysis of these narratives, specifically focusing on the relationship between immigrant parents and their 'left behind children,' we have managed to depict how deeply affected these children, now adults, are by the early and prolonged separation from their parents. In fact, we feel that their experience could be described as what Terr (1994) calls Type 2 trauma, taking place over a long period of time within the silence of a family or of society. For we fear that these children's stories have not been thoroughly heard; and when children's voices are not heard in the family or outside, that may result to a vicarious traumatization, which might be even more serious than the original act (Mucci, 2013). We strongly believe that psychoanalytic research and practice are capable of bearing witness to what in society is in danger of undergoing repression and marginalization (ibid). The present research is a tentative attempt to this direction.

When narrating their stories, the participants often told us that this is a painful subject for them, and their emotional reactions attested to that. The interviews were equally demanding on the countertransference level. Primo Levi (2015) distinguishes traumatized people into two categories: those who talk and those who remain silent. Those who remain silent are often condemned to a dehydrated existence. However, the narrative also involves risks of reactivating the trauma, triggering shame and terror (Rosenblum, 2009). We believe that the interviews with the participants produced narratives that were able to capture their experience and meaning making of it, while also providing the participants a 'safe space' where they could process their experience. Thus, they managed to turn this absence into a story: a story, quite similar to the story Ulysses narrated to the Phaeacians, about separation, abandonment, and loss.[2]

Notes

1 Data deriving from the 2011 population census by the National Greek Statistical Service.
2 A psychoanalytic and qualitative research on immigrants' 'left-behind' children: "I understand why they left, but why did they leave?" (Anagnostaki & Zaharia, 2020).

References

Ainsworth, M. D. S., Blehar, M. C., Waters, E., & Wall, S., Patterns of Attachment: Psychological Study of the Strange Situation. Hillsdale, NJ: Erlbaum, 1978.

Akhtar, S., Immigration and Acculturation: Mourning, Adaptation, and the Next Generation. New York, NY: Aronson, 2011.

Akhtar, S., Immigration and Identity: Turmoil, Treatment, and Transformation. Northvale, NJ: Aronson, 1999.

Anagnostaki, L., & Zaharia A., A Psychoanalytic and Qualitative Research on Immigrants' "Left-Behind" Children: "I Understand Why They Left, But Why Did They Leave?" International Journal of Applied Psychoanalytic Studies, 1–15, 2020. DOI: 10.1002/aps.1646

Antman, F. M., Gender, Educational Attainment, and The Impact of Parental Migration on Children Left Behind. Journal of Population Economics, 25, 1187–1214, 2012. DOI: 10.1007/s00148-012-0423-y

Arnold, E., Separation and Loss through Immigration of African Caribbean Women to UK. Attachment and Human Development, 8, 159–174, 2007. DOI: 10.1080/14616730600789472

Arnold, E., Working with Families of African Caribbean Origin: Understanding Issues around Immigration and Attachment. London: Jessika Kingsley Publications, 2011.

Bernardi, R., What Kind of Discipline Is Psychoanalysis? The International Journal of Psychoanalysis, 96, 731–754, 2015. DOI: 10.1111/1745-8315.12351

Bohleber, W., Remembrance, Trauma and Collective Memory. The Battle for Memory in Psychoanalysis. The International Journal of Psychoanalysis, 88, 329–352, 2007. DOI: 10.1516/V5H5-8351-7636-7878

Bowlby, J., Attachment and Loss, Vol. 1. Attachment. London: Penguin Books, 1969.

Brearley, M., Social Trauma. In E. McGinley, & A. Varchevker (Eds.), Enduring Trauma Through the Life Cycle. London: Karnac Books, 2013.

Dreby, J., Divided by Borders: Mexican Migrants and Their Children. Los Angeles: University of California Press, 2010.

Erikson, K. T., Everything in its Path. New York, NY: Simon and Schuster, 1976.

Freud, S., Beyond the Pleasure Principle, S. E. 18: 1–6, 1920.

Freud, S., Inhibitions, Symptoms and Anxiety, S. E. 20: 77–174, 1926.

Gallant T. W., Modern Greece: From the War of Independence to the Present. 2nd Edition. London: Bloomsbury, 2016.

Garland, C., Thinking about Trauma. In C. Garland (Ed.), Understanding Trauma: A Psychoanalytical Approach. Tavistock Clinic Series. London: Duckworth, 1998.

Graham, E., & Jordan, L., Migrant Parents and the Psychological Well-being of Left-behind Children in Southeast Asia. Journal of Marriage and Family, 73, 763–87, 2011. DOI: 10.1111/j.1741-3737.201.00844.x

Greenberg, J. & Mitchell, S. A., Object Relations in Psychoanalytic Theory. Cambridge: Cambridge University Press, 1983.

Grinberg, L. & Grinberg, R., Psychoanalytic Perspectives on Migration and Exile. London: Yale University Press, 1989.

Gurevich, H., The Language of Absence. International Journal of Psychoanalysis, 89, 561–578, 2008.

Hirschberger, G., Collective Trauma and the Social Construction of Meaning. Frontiers in Psychology, 9: 1441, 2018. DOI: 10.3389/fpsyg.2018.01441

Holpuch, A., Families divided at the border: The most horrific immigration policy I've ever seen. The Guardian. Retrieved from http//www.theguardian.com, 2018.

Homer, The Odyssey. Athens: Manolis Triantafyllidis Foundation, 2009.

Kaplan, S., Children in Genocide. Extreme Traumatization and the 'Affect Propeller'. The International Journal of Psychoanalysis, 87, 725–746, 2006. DOI: 10.1516/9C86-H1RG-K3FF-DRAH

Kotzamanis, V., & Mihos, Z., Pou Gennithika, Pou Katoiko? H Geographiki Kinitikotita ston Elladiko Choro: Mia Prtoti Choriki Proseggisi [Where Was I Born, Where Do I Live? Geographical Mobility in Greece: Attempt for a Spatial Approach]. Volos: Laboratory of Demographic and Social Analyses of University of Thessalia, 2005.

Laub, D., & Auerhahn, N. C., Failed Empathy: A Central Theme in the Survivor's Holocaust Experience. Psychoanalytic Psychology, 6, 377–400, 1989. DOI: 10.1037/0736-9735.6.4.377

Lazaretou, S., "Figi anthropinou kefalaiou: Sinchroni tasi metanastefsis ton Ellinon sta chronia tis krisis." ["Flight of Human Resources: The Modern Trend of Immigration of Greeks in the Time of Crisis."] Financial Report of the Bank of Greece, 4, 33–58, 2016.

Levi, P., The Complete Works of Primo Levi. New York, NY: Norton & Co., 2015.

Midgley, N. Sailing between Scylla and Charybdis: Incorporating Qualitative Approaches into Child Psychotherapy Research. Journal of Child Psychotherapy, 30, 89–111, 2004. DOI: 10.1080/0075417042000205814

Midgley, N., Psychoanalysis and Qualitative Psychology: Complementary or Contradictory Paradigms? Qualitative Research in Psychology, 3, 1–19, 2006. DOI: 10.1191/1478088706qrp065oa

Mucci, C., Beyond Individual and Collective Trauma: Intergenerational Transmission, Psychoanalytic Treatment, and the Dynamics of Forgiveness. London: Karnac Books, 2013.

Näslund, B., Persson-Blennow, I., McNeil, T., Kaij, L., & Malmquist-Larsson, A., Offspring of Women with Nonorganic Psychosis: Infant Attachment to the Mother at One Year. Acta Psychiatrica Scandinavica, 69, 231–241, 1984.

Recalcati, M., Il Complesso di Telemaco: Genitori e Figli dopo il Tramonto del Padre [The Complex of Telemachus: Parents and Children after the Father's Sunset]. Rome: Anagrama, 2015.

Rosenblum, R., Postponing Trauma: The Dangers of Telling. International Journal of Psychoanalysis, 90, 1319–1340, 2009.

Rosnik, P. (Reporter), Mental Pain and Social Trauma. The International Journal of Psychoanalysis, 94, 1200–1202, 2013. DOI: 10.1111/1745-8315.12165

Rustin, M., Migration and creativity. In A. Varchevker, & E. McGinley (Eds.), Enduring Migration through the Life Cycle. London: Karnac Books, 2013.

Shamani, M., Is Poverty a Collective Trauma? A Joint Learning Process with Women Living in Poverty in the City of Haifa in Israel. The British Journal of Social Work, 48, 1718–1735, 2018. DOI: 10.1093/bjsw/bcx116

Shear, M. D., Goodnough, A., & Haberman, M., Trump retreats on separating families, but thousands may remain apart. *The New York Times*, 2018. Retrieved from http//www.nytimes.com

Smith, J. A. (2011). Evaluating the Contribution of Interpretative Phenomenological Analysis. Health Psychology Review, 5, 9–27, 2011. DOI: 10.1080/17437199.2010.510659

Smith, J. A., & Eatough, V., Interpetative Phenomenological Analysis. In A. Coyle, & E. Lyons (Eds.), Analysing Qualitative Data in Psychology. London: Sage, 2007.

Smith, J. A., Flowers, P., & Larkin, M., Interpretative Phenomenological Analysis: Theory, Method and Research. London: Sage, 2009.

Suarez-Orozco, C., Todorova, L.G., & Louie, J., Making Up for Lost Time: The Experience of Separation and Reunification Among Immigrant Families. Family Process, 41, 625–643, 2002.

Terr, L., Unchained Memories: True Stories of Traumatic Memories, Lost and Found. New York, NY: Basic Books, 1994.

Varchenvker, A., Introduction. In A. Varchevker, & E. McGinley (Eds.), Enduring Migration through the Life Cycle. London: Karnac Books, 2013.

Volkan, V. D., Immigrants and Refugees: Trauma, Perennial Mourning, Prejudice, and Border Psychology. London: Karnac Books, 2017.

Volkan, V. V., Nostalgia as a Linking Phenomenon. Journal of Applied Psychoanalytic Studies, 1, 169–179, 1999.

Wen, M., & Lin, D., Child Development in Rural China: Children Left Behind by Their Migrant Parents and Children on Nonmigrant Families. Child Development, 83, 120–136, 2011. DOI: 10.1111/j.1467-8624.2011.01698.x

Yang, Y., The Impact of Psychic Trauma on Individualization and Self-identity: How the Psychic Trauma of Poverty Affects Individuation and Self-identity in the Context of Chinese Family. In D. E. Scharff, & S. Varvin (Eds.), Psychoanalysis in China. Manila: Phoenix Publishing House, 2014.

Chapter 12

Subtle Paths of Trauma in Migrating Families

Daniela Lucarelli and Ludovica Grassi

Adolescence and migration are catastrophic changes from known to unknown and from sameness to otherness. They deeply affect the family skin envelope and its permeability and integrity, by setting in motion a renegotiation of the narcissistic contract between subjects and groups endorsed at birth with the belonging community. The narcissistic contract establishes the bond of filiation through the acknowledgement of the newborn as a member of the group by the *whole*, and of his family and social group as his origin by the child, who commits to carry on their models, meanings and legacy. According to Aulagnier (1975), the narcissistic contract, signed by the child and the group, results from the pre-investment by the *whole* of the place that the *subject* is supposed to occupy in the future and of the *infant* itself as a future voice that will perpetuate the group's sociocultural model. The subject's identity is therefore built up at the intersection of the possible perpetuity of the group with the individual's desire of perpetuity, grounded in a narcissistic wish for immortality. In return for his investment onto the group and its models, the child will get the right to occupy an independent place from just the parental discourse and judgement, the illusion of a timeless persistency projected onto the *whole* and the access to a historical dimension. As a result, he will be able to develop his own *identificatory project*, that amounts to what the "I" *hopes* to become, a hope that needs to be valued both by the subject and by the group.

When there is a conflict or a rupture between the parental couple and its environment, the risk arouses confirmation of the children's phantasies of rejection, exclusion, aggression and omnipotence. More specifically, migrations problematically affect filiation processes, as a result of experiences of conception, pregnancy, delivery and early infant care occurring outside the original cultural and affective environment: parents-to-be are in fact deprived of most of their socio-cultural systems of reference, that are essential to work out such experiences. The very possibility to appoint the child the role of descendant, namely to engage him in a symbolic filiation made of intertwined ancestries and sense of belonging, is jeopardized.

DOI: 10.4324/9781003269649-17

Both adolescents and migrants feel, for a long time, suspended between two worlds, no more there, not yet here. A space-time rupture marks both the experiences, wherein a pivotal role is played by the body that is affected both in its perception and its meaning. Moreover, in migrating families there is quite often a deep dislocation of the place that the adolescent occupies or could have occupied in the family ensemble. A distortion of the subject's historicization and identificatory project are hence at play in different ways in each member of the family. During adolescence, pubertal turmoil may have a disorganizing effect upon the mind and raise confusional and depressive anxieties, resulting in troubles of identification processes. In addition, since identity building is intertwined with social and cultural identity, as well as to filiation movements, their upsetting or distress affects the subject's inclination to either blur or stiffen his identity boundaries, possibly resulting in violence or other kinds of antisocial behaviours, up to extreme solutions such as murderous and violent acts, both self- and other-directed.

The unfolding of acculturation and affiliation processes in individuals and families are intersubjective in nature and deeply affected by the host society. The balance between filiation and affiliation is subverted both in adolescence and in migration: in the migration experience, the whole family and its members are involved because of the need to resume affiliation processes, which can be dramatically difficult when impressive or subtler traumatic experiences undermine the basic trust in a supporting internal object. In adolescence, significant difficulties of affiliation processes may occur due to an excessive gap between what is familiar and what is stranger: the adolescent may feel he is losing his own identity and a sense of continuity of his own self. Different outcomes, such as integration, assimilation, rejection or withdrawal may surface into the first as well as second and third generation, by means of complex inter- and trans-generational dynamics.

Violeta and Her Family

The whole family enters my office for the first meeting, which Lisa, the mother, requested by phone. On that occasion, she pointed at the 17-year-old daughter as the reason for the couple's request for psychotherapy, due to her accusation against the step-father Adrian for sexual abuse. In such a family setting, Violeta breaks through as the one who embodies trauma, violence and excess and challenges the basic links of the family and its horizontal and vertical boundaries. That's why group settings, and especially family settings, are specifically designed to deal with traumatic pathologies, as they are equipped to detect and work upon boundary sufferings, both at a spatial and temporal level. Violeta appears immediately to be a key element in the family, in its history, myths and links. Although the mother's request is for couple psychotherapy, I feel that all the expectation is focused on Violeta, who arrives very calmly at my office, stopping to play with and cuddle a cat sitting along my driveway.

Lisa starts off by the statement that they come from L, a pretty remote district in our city. Then she addresses our focus onto Violeta, whom she qualifies as problematic. *Last year she ran away from home, so I went to the Police and was told to take her to the police station when she would show up again. So did I: at that time she reported that my husband, who is not her biologic father, seven years before had touched her. Now there is an ongoing judicial proceeding. She is on psychotherapy, but her attendance is erratic. Nobody in the family has been banished.*

After her mother's inception, Violeta spontaneously steps in: *I don't know what to think. Maybe I am nuts…but I am convinced it is true… maybe he did it accidentally. Earlier we were like this (nodding to her step-father and tying up two fingers). I still love him. But sometimes I make a scene, whilst I used to be a quiet person. Yet his answer is always that one, he never caved in. I would not tell if I weren't sure.*

The younger brother, in disagreement with Violeta, states that he was the first to be told by her of the abuse: he felt uncertain, doubtful because of the seven years elapsed. Eventually, he realized he couldn't believe it.

The father is silent. When urged on, he only tells that everything was fine before.

In this immigrant family, the daughter's adolescence violently brings to the fore, as in *après coup*, all the traumatic experiences that are inherent in migration as well as in the transgenerational flow pertaining both to the family and to their home country. However, the father's *"before"* tells us that this family's time is torn into a *before* and an *after,* which results in the asphyxia of the dynamic time of *après coup*, as it is stiffened in such static duality. The father's charge dates back seven years, more or less immediately after the family setting in the new country, that followed a long separation of the children from the father and recurring shorter separations from the mother. But in the past, there was also a separation from Violeta's natural father, when Lisa was five-months pregnant: a slap in the face accounted for Lisa's firm resolution to divorce. The low severity of the alleged facts (a slap and a touching, both occurring once) needs to be matched with the experience of an alcoholic father on the mother's part and a father who died when Adrian was coming of age. The violent father was also embodied in the ruthless dictator ruling, until recently, the home country, whose loss of power is now regretted because of the greater safety felt under his regime and better keeping of borders; now all the family members are scattered all over the world. Moreover, the family boundaries have now been invaded by socio-health services alerted by the police and the court.

Even in the original families there is a remarkable dislocation: the nationality is the same in both families, but they belong to several different language and cultural groups. Among the many languages spoken within this family, the kids chose the Italian, claiming it is *easier*, despite they came to Italy at 7 and 5 years of age, respectively. The dislocated narcissistic contract is not the same for all the family members.

Resuming the idea of similarity between adolescence and migration, both implying a reorganization of a narcissistic contract and involving a specific psychic function, we want to emphasize that they also entail an *in-between* position that, at best, is characterized by a transitional quality with an open and movable boundary and coexistence of either conflicting or coming and going elements. Nostalgia is an appropriate illustration of this intermediate area, as well as its function of linking past and present, original and adoption countries, filiation and affiliation... In this family, the mother is positioned *between* her husband and her daughter, *between* the time of Violeta's report and of the inherent facts, and *between* different geographical places and languages. However, there is no place for nostalgia, because the very transitional dimension is lacking: the *in-between* puts irreconcilable alternatives, demanding splits and mutilations of parts of reality and experience. Any vital impulse is restrained in a deadly grip that prevents psychic work and the dealing with otherness and change: both mother and her husband gave up the effort to understand the meaning of Violeta's late allegation against her step-father and the concomitant alienation from family life (Violeta spends most nights outside home, by friends Lisa and Adrian neither know, nor try to get in touch with). She often does not answer her mobile phone, therefore even her mother's feeble attempts to hear from her come to nothing. Giulian, Violeta's brother and the only child of the current couple, embodies his parents' expectation of a well-adapted son, who does not arouse thoughts and worries in his conforming to a neutral model of behaviour, that is reasonable both in Italy and in their original country.

All psychic work is in abeyance, as well as memory and expectations, frozen and lifeless, clinging to concreteness, with the couple fiercely keeping their feet on the ground: maybe it is not by chance that the father works as a floor layer and the mother as a scrubwoman who, accordingly, cleans floors. Rejection and defence against thinking and symbolizing date back to a sequence of traumatic experiences: from the dictatorship in the original country, through the personal experiences in the families of origin with their incumbencies, up to migration and eventually the current family situation. Shame, violence and the imposition of silence result in narcissistic gaps where representation and words are not admitted: this is conveyed to the succeeding generations, as we can see in a dearth of language and phantasy in this family, notwithstanding the plurality of languages spoken in the original families. Significantly, the young generation chooses Italian as *the easiest* among all the available languages, as a defensive manic move of adaptation, aimed at obliterating an inadmissible depression rooted in the original world, turned thereby into something stranger: *over there it is boring*. As an adolescent, Violeta is undertaking a migration through different life stages, bonds and languages, that prevents her feeling at home either here or there. But the unresolved issues inherent to her family context pushed her to take on the task of expressing, on behalf of all family members, the exile, the abandonment of original bonds, the rupture of social and cultural links, the fading of boundaries and, moreover, the unmetabolizable sexual excess, the traumatic potential and the prevented integration.

In spite of the court, of social services, of psychologists and so on, this family will probably never succeed in achieving a shared truth, which in fact would need a good enough attitude to psychic work and linking activity.

Karima's Tears

Karima's parents Kamal and Meriam, originating from North Africa, come to the clinic of a psychotherapy association claiming that their second-born Karima, a 12-year-old, is lately assailed by intense anxiety that she expresses through endless crying, restlessness, tremor and nosebleed. Sleep is troubled, too: she cannot fall asleep alone and often wakes up in the grip of nightmares or pavor nocturnus.

Before the first meeting, there is an impressive call to the therapist, whom the family does not know yet. In this phone call Kamal anxiously begs the therapist to talk with his daughter, without considering how whim is this request, but expressing a need of absolute trust and dependence: the unknown therapist is supposed to be endowed with the containing ability that he lacks and that can receive and hold Karima's suffering. Something irrepressible and unthinkable appears to break through boundaries from the daughter to the father and, now, to the therapist. Though the astonished therapist replies she is willing to meet them all, but she can't help Karima right now, having never got to know her, Kamal hands the phone to her addressing the therapist: "You do have to talk with her, she feels too bad!"

The therapist, now on the phone with the crying girl who screams unintelligible words, experiences unsettling feelings: she feels emotionally engaged but, at the same time, a stranger who knows nothing. She looks for words to voice her recognition of Karima's pain and her will to share it when they will meet, but the girl keeps crying in despair, while firmly clinging to the phone, with the father doing nothing to stop this situation. The therapist, by activating her holding and empathizing abilities, finds herself suggesting to try breathing together, smoother and smoother, while setting the pace of breath. Little by little, Karima calms down, and agrees to say good-bye to the therapist and to wait for their forthcoming meeting.

This is a very intriguing and unique incident, where the sensorial component of breathing is predominant and becomes an early link between patient and therapist: holding and containment occur at a sensorial level. Later, during a session, Karima will emphasize how beautiful was the therapist's voice, one more sensorial element. As in Violeta's case, we are dealing with poor and torn subjects' and family's boundaries, that let emotions overflow and violate the therapist's boundaries. We are moved by the therapist's opposite feelings of closeness and alienness in resonance with the difficult integration of sameness and otherness, and of belonging and exclusion from the home country and the host country as well. A known and close person was unable to perform the needed reassuring function, which was assigned, therefore, to a distant and unknown person: distance and closeness do not complement each other, being confused instead. Accordingly, in the succeeding sessions, a denial of feelings of estrangement due to migration will emerge, as well as conditions of inordinate closeness between father and daughter, thus obliterating generational differences and separateness between different family members. As is often the case in migration vicissitudes, reality confronts the subject with the double, that is the background of all psychic facts: double country, double language, double culture and binomial pairs such as near-faraway, included-excluded, internal-external, welcomed-rejected and same-different. The therapist is left wondering about this family's attitude to carry out the psychic work required to integrate these elements and thereby enrich the members' Egos.

> Karima asks to see alone the therapist, and her parents, who accompany her, anxiously voice their and her high expectations of this meeting. The evaluation involves sessions with the girl, with the couple and with the family. During her first session, Karima reports her anxiety and sleeping difficulties. By recently studying at school the reproductive system, she has better understood how sexuality works between a couple: after witnessing intimate warmth between her parents (kisses, hugs in bed), she began feeling extremely anxious when it becomes dark, being incapable to handle the idea of intimacy between her parents. This account proceeds on and off: flood of words, tears, silences, smiles and then all over again. Parents seem to have lost the distance that allowed them to function as a protective shield since the infantile Oedipal organization, and to have become instead a source of excitation through resexualization of links.
>
> The couple's history is marked by many separations that make up the leitmotiv of the relationship. Both partners are last-born children, after more than ten siblings, and are born in different towns in the same country. They met in a taxi, an apt representation of an intermediate element but also of being in abeyance between two alterities. As customary in their culture, they married in one month. Soon after, during

> the first pregnancy, Kamal moves to Italy to begin a work activity, while Meriam stays at home to take care of their first-born girl. There is a two-year separation, that according to Meriam was not painful, since she kept feeling her husband affectively close to both her and Karima, who was fully aware that he was her father.

This account outlines a relatedness built inside a fusional system that finds expression through absolute, all-encompassing categories, such as goodness, safety, trust: being a whole, distances can be denied. Maybe such defensive organization results from a poor internal world with regard to introjected good primary objects: both partners were presumably entrusted to the care of older siblings rather than of their exhausted mothers. Migration is described as without rips or strains, though there is a mother left alone while giving birth and raising her first baby, who after two years agrees to move to an unknown country without either perplexity or fear. Karima is the first child born in the new country, where the family experienced several transfers before settling down. Karima was a precocious girl, starting to talk very early, in Italian too. On the other hand, she experienced separation anxieties, particularly from the father, during preschool and primary school, resulting in a difficult integration into the school environment. Karima and her elder sister speak fluent Italian and Arabic, that is the shared language at home, whereas the youngest boy, affected by a speech disorder, cannot speak Arabic at all.

What stands out in this situation is an attitude toward normalization and flattening of emotions through an avoiding and denial of thought, pain and distress. Feelings of uprooting and nostalgia, typical in migrants, do not surface, while we observe a pseudo-adaptation and an apparent assimilation of the new culture that require a split of a part of the self (Eiguer, 2017). The children's symptoms express the pain of the whole family, representing exclusion and an unthinkable separation trauma. The parents try to make the family a shelter from the outside world as, for example, by keeping Karima's adolescent sister from going out with peers, thereby stifling her attraction toward the world of otherness.

The consultation itself bursts into the family, similarly to the symmetrical family's invasion of the therapist's boundaries, giving presence to unthinkable and uncontrollable experiences, in the absence of psychic tools to contain and process them. The onset of puberty (Gutton, 1991), for Karima, is the confusion of languages and experiencing a violent sexual excitation, introduced by adults, without protective shields and translating codes (Laplanche, 1980). As for Violeta, the adults' passion has become the child's, while the need of psycho-somatic caring has grown out of proportion. Adolescents deal with a new language and are in search of answers from adults. Sexuality is pivotal not only because of changes during puberty, but as a crucible of most secrets of life, of origins and of the why of things

(De Simone, 2009). Puberty brings about the unfathomable leap of experiencing one's own sexualized body, which re-signifies everything. What was well known and predictable is now hyper-exciting and/or bewildering: the parents and their bodies, the Oedipal issues and identifications, one's own identity of being a child of those specific parents, phantasies about origins of psychic functioning and individual rather than generational myths as the foundation of subjectivity: in other words, a true re-edition of the narcissistic contract.

As psychic life springs from a loss and the never-extinguished wish to fill up the resulting gap, to reunite body and spirit, "the sexual is there, wherever life tries to regenerate from that cleavage" (Algini, 2001). Both for Karima and Violeta, the onset of puberty opened a break between the lost childhood and the need to deal with the intensity of drives and the strife of building an identificatory project; moreover, identifications are not easy, due to their parents' frailty in their sense of identity and belonging, and to unrepresentable traumatic experiences dug in the family history. Opening up to adolescence involves being able to abandon the infantile omnipotence and to move from a narcissistic dual relatedness up to a more mature ability to bear ambivalence and, as a result, to mourn. On the contrary, Karima cannot acknowledge her parents' sexual link and keeps the idea of an absolute possession of both them, while Violeta clings to her Oedipal relationship, positioning herself between her mother and step-father. They cannot deal with the dreadful knowledge of the real nature of parents' relationship and of the Oedipal triangle. A "relationship of a third kind" (Britton, 1989), wherein the subject is not included, cannot be experienced, maybe for the failed achievement of Bion's third element of psychic life: K or Knowledge.

As described in Violeta's family predicament, Karima uncovers a deadlock "in-between" situation, unfit to develop into a transitional area: the taxi where the parents met is still running around without a destination. In the same way as her parents could not experience an intermediate time between meeting and marrying, so transitions are very troublesome for her, pushed forward by her infantile precociousness and now by adolescent fantasies and the peer group pull, but at the same time turned around to regressive needs that were not met in due time. In both cases, we are confronted with bumpy rides of the last generation's identity processes and projects: they are affected by loads and frailties descending from ancestors' unelaborated traumas and more extensive socio-historical conditions.

The family setting allows itself to host and hold painful issues that are rooted in preceding generations, as well as to witness, in the concreteness of family exchanges, the quality of individual and group somato-psychic functioning and the hold and attitude to psychic work by the subject's and family's boundaries or skin. These are all elements specifically put under stress by migratory vicissitudes, that always involve a significant traumatic value. The adolescent as well as the stranger can be viewed as specific detectors of social and cultural faults, contradictions and weaknesses, triggering in the human surroundings resistances that require new semiotic and interpreting instruments to be overcome.[1]

Note

1 A paper on a similar theme was published in Le Divan familial, no 44/2020.

References

Algini, M. L., Il Sessuale, Borla, Roma, 2001.
Aulagnier, P., La violence de interprétation. Du pictogramme à l'énoncé. PUF, Paris, 1975.
Britton, R., The missing link: Parental Sexuality in the Oedipus Complex, in The Oedipus Complex today, ed. J. Steiner, Karnaac Books, London, 1989.
De Simone, G., Edipo e la conoscenza, in Campanile P. (a cura di) Parricidio e Figlicidio crocevia d'Edipo, Borla, Roma, 2008.
Eiguer, A., La difference culturelle et l'étrangeté dans la famille migrante, Le Divan Familial, 2017/1, InPress, Paris, 2017.
Gutton, P.,"Quadrige" PUF, Paris, 1991.
Laplanche, J., Nouveaux fondements pour la psychanalyse, PUF, Paris, 1980.

Part V

Posttraumatic Conditions

New Theoretical and Clinical Approach

Chapter 13

Psychotherapy of Posttraumatic Conditions

Sverre Varvin, Tija Despotovic, and Vladimir Jović

Introduction

Refugees flee from war, persecution, torture and other human rights violations (HRV), many meeting extreme conditions during their flight with maltreatment (including by police and border guards), rape, death and extreme insecurity (Jović, 2018). Many become severely traumatized suffering complicated losses with little or no possibility to mourn them.

Many have been exposed to undefined waiting during flight and when arriving in a country where they can seek asylum. Waiting is often experienced as a great mental pressure (Sagbakken, Bregård and Varvin, 2020). Western countries have now developed strategies of deterrence with strict border controls and policies aiming at keeping refugees away (Gammeltoft-Hansen, 2016; Weber, 2017).

Research has shown an overrepresentation of mental health suffering among individuals with a refugee background compared to the majority population (Fazel, Wheeler and Danesh, 2005; Priebe *et al.*, 2010; Fazel *et al.*, 2012; Sabes-Figuera *et al.*, 2012; Bogic, Njoku and Priebe, 2015; Hocking, Kennedy and Sundram, 2015; Hassan *et al.*, 2016), even after many years in a host country (Vaage *et al.*, 2010; Opaas, Wentzel-Larsen and Varvin, 2020). There is high degree of resilience among refugees (Sleijpen *et al.*, 2016; UNHCR, 2016), which is highly dependent on possibilities for treatment and for making a decent life (Ungar, 2012; Betancourt *et al.*, 2015; Varvin, 2015). Children (slightly less than half of displaced persons), mothers with children, elders and torture survivors are among the most vulnerable. Their basic needs and health care needs are often insufficiently covered and traumatized refugees regularly wait for years before they get adequate treatment, if at all (Opaas and Varvin, 2015).

The main aim of this chapter is to contribute to the understanding of the impact of traumatic experiences with disruption of psychological functions, such as capacity for symbolization and affect regulation and the consequences of halted mourning processes.

DOI: 10.4324/9781003269649-19

The aim of psychoanalytic psychotherapy is directed at unlocking developmental arrests, helping patients with difficult mourning processes and repairing effects of regression and the disruptive potential of annihilation anxieties. In this context, we will analyse how posttraumatic sequelae are conceptualized in modern academic psychiatry and then develop the advantage of a psychoanalytical approach and describe how psychoanalytic treatment may work for this often severely traumatized group of people. We illustrate it with two clinical case presentations, the first of one refugee in individual psychotherapy in Norway and the second as excerpts of group analytical psychotherapy in Serbia in times of war.

Conceptualization of Posttraumatic States: Model of PTSD

Current conceptualization of posttraumatic sequelae is encircled and almost synonymous of posttraumatic stress disorder (PTSD), conceptualized in 1980. At that time, it was needed and it helped to formulate the suffering of large groups of traumatized individuals, but with time, shortcomings of the type of diagnostic system it was built on have come to the fore.

It was conceived as a revolutionary restructuring of psychiatric methodology (Mayes and Horwitz, 2005), which brought to life a "syndromal nosology" in the third edition of the "Diagnostic and Statistical Manual of Mental Disorders," or DSM-III (American Psychiatric Association, 1980). DSM-III represented a significant deviation from previous versions in that it introduced: 1) explicit diagnostic criteria; 2) a multi-axial system; and 3) a descriptive approach that pretended to be neutral *vis-à-vis* etiological theories ("atheoretical"). Mental disorders were now defined as syndromes or as clusters of symptoms that appear together. Later it was recognized "that the DSM has been explicitly atheoretical but implicitly a medical model" (Follette and Houts, 1996); the main assumption was that mental disorders should be explained by changes at the structure or molecular functions of the brain. It brought fundamental conflict from within: mental disorders were defined as illnesses (in a framework of the biomedical model), but conceptualized according to behavioural analysis (i.e. signs and symptoms that are, in their essence, the patient's statements or actions).

The historical accounts describing the process of designing PTSD (Young, 1995; Shephard, 2001), show an interesting collaboration between clinicians and researchers that resulted in this kind of model for posttraumatic sequelae. A precursor was the description of the "Post-Vietnam syndrome" in a 1972 article in *The New York Times* written by Chaim Shatan (1972), a practicing psychoanalyst who was working with self-help groups for war veterans. The development of conceptualizations of a posttraumatic syndrome changed significantly with the introduction of the "information processing model," by Mardi Horowitz (Young, 1995).

This descriptive approach has had many unwanted consequences, first being the overall reduction of descriptive power; this strategy of relying on behavioural analysis only, i.e. checking for appearance of specific signs and symptoms (statements or changes in behaviour), can exclude many aspects of the clinical picture that could be important for our understanding of posttraumatic sequelae. Probably the most illustrative example is the inclusion, and then very fast exclusion, of the feeling of guilt in the diagnostic criteria for PTSD: although it had been listed in criterion D in DSM-III ("*guilt about surviving when others have not, or about behaviour required for survival*" [American Psychiatric Association, 1980]), it was excluded from DSM-III-R. As we know from our clinical work, there is no traumatic experience without some degree of reflections of the subject relating his/her own acts or failures that are somehow connected to feelings of guilt and responsibility. But at the same time, guilt feelings are extremely painful, and survivors are very often compelled to cope with them through powerful defence mechanisms such as dissociation or denial.

Probably even more important were consequences of this conceptualization with its focus on cognitive processes and memory function, to understanding of therapeutic approach. As a traumatic memory was perceived as a main causative factor, many therapies were constructed with an aim to "reach" the memory and transform it; it focused on pathogenic effects of traumatic memory, which facilitated the development of "trauma-focused psychotherapies" as "the most highly recommended type of treatment for PTSD. 'Trauma-focused' means that the treatment focuses on the memory of the traumatic event or its meaning" (*PTSD Treatment Basics - PTSD: National Center for PTSD*, no date). It is claimed that trauma-focused psychotherapies with the strongest evidence are: prolonged exposure (PE), cognitive processing therapy (CPT), and eye-movement desensitization and reprocessing (EMDR) (*ibid.*).

Traumatization — Psychoanalytical Understanding

There is a wide range of symptoms and suffering after trauma that are not included into the description of PTSD. Traumatized persons struggle with mental and physical pain that is difficult to understand put into words. The pain may be expressed as dissociated states of mind, as bodily pain and other somatic experiences and dysfunctions, as overwhelming thoughts and feelings, as behavioral tendencies and relational styles or as ways of living and so forth. Further, the effects of severe and complicated losses (loss of close ones, loss of property, loss of culture and so forth), need to be understood as this is an important part of the experience of traumatized refugees (Nickerson *et al.*, 2014; Varvin, 2016). Traumatization may be a causative and/or disposing factor in many psychopathological manifestations: depression, addiction, eating disorders, personality dysfunctions and anxiety states (Taft *et al.*, 2007; Vitriol *et al.*, 2009; Purnell, 2010; Vaage *et al.*, 2010; Leuzinger-Bohleber, 2012).

Being traumatized is an experience of something unexpected that should not happen. It creates an internal situation of profound helplessness and an experience of being abandoned by all good and helping persons and internal objects. The feeling of helplessness and being abandoned may be carried over into the posttraumatic phase. A deep fear of an impending catastrophe of helplessness where nobody will help or care may develop. An inner feeling of desperation and fear of psychosomatic breakdown with fear of annihilation may ensue and much of posttraumatic pathology may be seen as a defence against and an attempt to cope with this impending catastrophe (Laub and Podell, 1995; Freedman *et al.*, 2018).

What is common are deficiencies in the representational system related to traumatic and other experiences; these experiences are painfully felt and set their marks on the body and the mind but are poorly contained in the mind. They are either not or deficiently symbolized in the sense that they cannot be expressed in narratives in a way where meaning can emerge and be reflected upon. These remain in the mind as dissociated or encapsulated fragments that have a disturbing effect on mood and mental stability (Rosenbaum and Varvin, 2007).

As a rule, extreme or complex traumatization (like rape or torture) eludes meaning when it happens and it precludes forming an internal third position where the person, in his or her own mind, can create a reflective distance to what is happening. The inner witnessing function, so vital for making meaning of experiences, is attacked during such extreme experiences, hindering the individual from being able to experience on a symbolic level the cruelties they have experienced.

The main mechanism that defines the strength of the Ego is a capacity for symbolization and mentalization, i.e. the capacity to transform raw sensory data (beta-elements), linking them to previous experience, understandings and concepts. This could be observed through a higher quality of associations and verbalizations as well as better affective modulation and eventually to "the emergence of mental contents and structures of increasingly higher levels of complexity, leading to symbolization and abstraction" (Lecours and Bouchard, 1997), p. 857. Observation that mentalization "absorbs internal as well as external stresses, traumatic excesses and internal pressures by mentally processing their effects on the soma/body and by elaborating these further" helps us to conceive this process as the "immune system" of the psyche (*ibid.*). When we say that ego-functions are destroyed in trauma, it is the equivalent of saying that its capacity to symbolize/mentalize is damaged, and it cannot produce layers of representations, which creates "a protective mental buffer formed from the successive layers of representations produced in the process of normal psychic development of the ego" (*ibid.*).

Psychoanalytic Treatment

How can people live through extreme and prolonged traumatization often in an extremely hostile environment and how do they organize their lives in the aftermath? Understanding these processes gives background to understanding how derivatives related to the traumatizing experiences manifest in the therapeutic process. A main point is that the analyst, when taking on the task of treating such traumatized patients, inevitably becomes involved in the not-symbolized, fragmentary and as a rule strongly affective scenarios related to the patient's traumatic experiences. This happens from the first encounter with the patient and is mostly expressed in the non-verbal interaction between the patient and the analyst. It may take a long time before these manifestations may be given a narrative form that, in a meaningful way, relates to traumatic and pre-traumatic experiences; it implies hard and painful emotional work from the patient, and from the analyst, to achieve this end (Sverre Varvin, 2013).

Several therapeutic approaches (e.g. EMDR, CBT (Cognitive Behaviour and Cognitive Processing)) focus on PTSD, depression and anxiety (Acarturk *et al.*, 2015; Wong *et al.*, 2015), so far with unconvincing results. Here we will focus on psychoanalytic treatment, a treatment many severely traumatized persons prefer (Van der Kolk and McFarlane, 1996). This user-based view on the advantages of psychoanalytic approaches was confirmed in research that demonstrated essential beneficiary aspects of psychodynamic therapy, as so-called evidence-based treatments had high drop-out and non-responder rates (Schottenbauer *et al.*, 2008) and showed benefits from psychodynamic therapies for the following reasons (*ibid.*):

- They address crucial areas in the clinical presentation of PTSD and the sequels of trauma that are not targeted by currently empirically supported treatments.
- They may be particularly helpful for complex PTSD as they target problems related to the self and self-esteem, ability to resolve reactions to trauma through improved reflective functioning and aim at the internalization of more secure inner working models of relationships.
- They work on improving social functioning.
- They show continued improvement after treatment ends.

For these not symbolized and insufficiently symbolized experiences to approach some integration and given some meaningful place in the individual's mind, they need to be actualized and given form in a holding and containing therapeutic relationship. This implies that the analyst must accept living with a patient in areas of the mind that are painfully absent of meaning and at times filled with horror. Further, without affirmation on the political, social and cultural level, the traumatized person's feeling of unreality and fragmentation connected with the experiences may continue as has been the case for many groups: Holocaust survivors, war veterans, victims of genocides etc. (Varvin, 2017).

One salient task in psychotherapy with traumatized patients is to enhance a metacognitive or mentalizing capacity that can enable the patient to deal more effectively with traces and derivatives of the traumatic experience. This implies helping the patient out of mental states characterized by concreteness and lack of dimensionality.

The task of therapy is to allow these poorly mentalized experiences to emerge in the transference relationship so that words and meaning can be co-created even if the experiences themselves by all human standards are cruel and devoid of meaning.

The traumatizing experiences must thus become actual in the therapeutic relationship. This may happen when the analyst is drawn into relational scenarios where he/she becomes part of the emerging trauma related scenes that the patient hitherto has struggled with alone.

Next, we will demonstrate one aspect of psychoanalytic therapy that may be an important step in this symbolizing process. We will especially focus on the therapeutic processes that deal with loss and postponed and complicated mourning. Loss may concern not only loss of close ones, of personal belongings, home, culture and home country, but there other dimensions of loss, including loss of basic safety, loss of bodily function and internal losses of the safety of the bond to the inner empathic object (Laub and Podell, 1995; Laub, 2005). Annihilation anxiety, which is predominant in traumatized persons, implies the fear of loss of self (Hurvich, 2003, 2015).

Loss and Trauma — A Case Story from Individual Psychoanalytic Psychotherapy

F, a woman in her late 30s, came to Norway as a refugee from a country in the Middle East nine years prior to treatment. She was in psychoanalytic psychotherapy face-to-face, twoo to three times a week, for a year and a half (this therapy analysis has been presented in Varvin and Stiles, 1999; Varvin, 2003).

She reported a relatively happy childhood. She was married and was working as clerk when she was arrested because of participating in a non-violent political organization together with her husband. At the time of her arrest, she was pregnant in the last trimester. She was maltreated physically (including beatings on her pregnant womb) and psychically (threats, seclusion etc.) and suffered from malnutrition and lack of proper medical care when she became ill. Her husband was arrested at the same time and was tortured to death some months later. She was allowed to go to a public hospital to give birth, and an escape was arranged for her shortly thereafter. While she was living clandestinely, her child died of an unknown disease, probably caused by the torture, maltreatment, and lack of adequate medical care during her stay in prison.

After the death of her child and husband, she lived in secret for about one year before she fled from her country under difficult circumstances. During this time, she experienced additional serious traumas.

She arrived in Norway severely depressed and suicidal and had serious eating problems in addition to post-traumatic and psychosomatic symptoms. In the years in Norway, she suffered almost continuously from nightmares, re-experiencing, avoidance behaviour, somatization and psychosomatic illness and recurrent depressions. Despite this, she managed to settle and achieve a considerable degree of integration in the community. She lived alone and had friends but no intimate contact with men. She had high levels of activity, lots of helping others, and little time for herself, seemingly reflecting a need to act rather than feel, characterized her life in exile.

F had to a large extent mourned her husband, for example, performing grief-rituals on his birthday. The loss of her child was not a problem she presented when seeking therapy and it remained silent during the first part until it emerged in a quite dramatic way in a session after a week's break in the treatment.

She arrived on time at the session, out of breath as she had been running believing she was late. Her first remark was. "I lost the bus" (a common expression in Norwegian when coming late for the bus, and here also indicating the theme of loss). In the first part of the session, she spoke in a staccato manner, evoking a strong need in the analyst to help and support her.

She talked about her loneliness during the break, the need to have someone to lean on, to trust and who could be close. The analyst affirmed her feeling of loneliness and her longing for a family. She then defended against this by idealizing a more independent life. Her own family and her close relations to them and also her ambivalent feelings toward them had been a theme throughout the therapy. In this section of the session, the analyst's interventions also became intellectual with a lack of affective resonance. The analyst did in this way join the patient in an enactment attempting to ward off painful material.

Then a shift occurred when the analyst remarked, remembering her earlier clearly stated affection for her family, that they, her family, surely would have liked her to establish a family in exile. She then became silent for some minutes and said crying:

"Yes, I have been thinking if I had my son, he would have been 10 years old and… "

She cried a lot and seemed distant, obviously re-experiencing scenes from the past. She then haltingly in short sentences, and after encouragement, talked about the birth of her child, how happy she had been when she heard the child cry. It felt like a victory. Also, the dangers came to her mind, and she was frightened and desperate in the session. She did not manage to stop crying as she left.

This was a breakthrough of memories, or rather a "recalling" or "evoking," which came as surprise for the patient (and for the analyst). It was a re-experiencing "like a film" of the trauma-scenario, a broken narrative.

She was physically ill during the night and when she came the next day, she was still quite affected. It gradually became clear what had happened before and during the previous sessions in fact represented an actualization of the drama when she lost her child.

Three consecutive nights before the key session she had had the following dream, which she told, realizing the connection with her child's death:

"And then suddenly I get all; I feel I, I got like; I had/I did not tell you, I dreamt for three nights [before the key session] that I cried. I was very narrow in my throat and, and had like saliva around my mouth. It's like a; then I thought like, what is it that makes me feel. I don't get enough oxygen and (heavy breathing), when I, eh, was in the middle of crying, when I woke up."

She was then able to tell how her child had died. At the time, she was in hiding and under poor living conditions. Her child got fever and had increasing difficulty breathing. In the end, the baby died in her arms of lack of air (asphyxia). Her despair and grief were abruptly interrupted by her dangerous circumstances, which demanded that she move on. Her baby was buried in haste and the harsh tone among her comrades stopped any attempt of her for emotional reactions.

We can now reconstruct aspects of what happened in her therapy. She had a markedly positive, almost idealizing transference toward the analyst. In the break, she had felt utmost loneliness, and this had evoked in her unconscious memories of her child as well as other persons she had lost (her husband and also her father when she was in exile). In the session, she came out of breath with a feeling of loss (expressed in her first remark: "I lost the bus"). The countertransference was characterized by a desperate wish to help, but then a feeling of helplessness that resulted in distancing and intellectualization on the analyst's side.

In hindsight, it was possible to identify several episodes earlier in the therapy where the theme of loss had come up and also where dead children had been mentioned. This had obviously been small attempts by the patient to bring maybe her most painful experience into the therapy, but she then backed away and either intellectualized or dropped the theme. The analyst had colluded with this and avoided the theme of loss, which had connection with the analyst's own problems and some unresolved issues concerning his own losses. These countertransference problems were possible to identify, understand and reflect on only when analysing the sessions afterward.

The theme of loss became, however, more acute for her in the break preceding this key-session. She had obviously during this time partly unconsciously lived through and been occupied with her tragic loss, identifying with her dead child and, by projective identification, the analyst got the role of the helpless helper that pushed him to act according to the role assigned to this part. This interpretation was supported by the analyst's subjective counter-transference reactions (i.e., feeling solicitous but helpless).

The relative abstinence in the session allowed her to start symbolizing her traumatic loss. The dreams were obviously a signal of an unconscious preparation for re-experiencing the death of her child in which she gave voice to the part of herself identified with the child trying to survive.

As the loss theme was elaborated, F began to integrate the loss of her child with her other losses — her husband's death, her father's death some years ago, and also other deaths. Thus, the emergence of the loss of her child brought with it memories of other losses, which she then worked to integrate and mourn during the rest of the therapy. She also had to face her guilt for not having been able to help her child, which may be interpreted as a survivor guilt.

Needless to say, this was a hard and laborious process for F and also for the analyst who had to work on his own unresolved issues. The work was completed and the treatment did make a difference in her life; she was no longer depressed and had less somatic pain and, more importantly, she started a new way of life. She was no longer the tireless helper; she took time to care for herself and relax and she managed to establish a relationship with a man.

F's experiences in her therapeutic process reflect complex interactions on a verbal and nonverbal level. Traumatic experiences are present in the mind and body of the traumatized in different ways, all seeking expression in communicative styles and ways of being in relation to the analyst. They may dramatically involve the analyst in processes that touch the analyst's own unresolved or partly resolved issues and draw him into a process of acting instead of thinking and reflecting. The transference-countertransference situation may push the analyst to become involved in a relational scenario that, as a rule, is possible to understand and interpret only after the fact. In the sequence presented from F's treatment, the analyst became the "helpless helper" in the transference and defended against this feeling by joining the patient's intellectualization. The transference situations vary, and different personas from the patient's internal world may appear in the transference as, for example, the perpetrator, the dehumanized victim and so forth.

It is argued that countertransference enactment may be a central vehicle for unsymbolized trauma-related material to emerge. When this happens, an opportunity may appear for the "unthought known" to be heard and contained in a joint created narrative that relates present suffering to past misery. A time-dimension can then be established in this area of the psyche, which also makes reflection possible. The precondition is attention to countertransference reactions and fantasies and the analyst's capacity for containment and gradual reflection and working though of the personal part of his reactions.

What happens is a mostly unconscious "*mise en scene*," which may happen over longer time in therapy. What we saw in this example was a more acute reaction of the analyst, but also that avoiding the loss theme probably had been going on for a prolonged part of the treatment.

Traumatized persons' experiences represent a partial foreclosure where parts of the symbolic function are undermined. Foreclosed signifiers are not integrated in the subject's unconscious so they tend to re-emerge from outside, in "the Real" (Lacan, 1977). Another way of saying this is that they appear as beta-elements and sometimes also as bizarre objects, experiences as coming from the outside through, for example, hallucinations (Bion, 1977). These mechanisms may also be reflected in traumatized persons' attention and concentration problems and their difficulties in organizing impressions in thoughts (Van der Kolk, 1994). Many traumatized persons have, moreover, experienced that language was perverted during torture and other atrocious situations; as a consequence they, to a large degree, have learned to rely on non-verbal communication. In torture, for example, everyday expressions are often used for the most gruesome torture practices, confusing communications are used to break down people and so forth.

The fact that so much of the focus in interpersonal relations with severely traumatized patients rely on the non-verbal dimensions may explain to a certain extent why many traumatized patients feel safe in a "psychoanalytic context" and why psychoanalytic therapy works when patient and analyst have different cultural backgrounds and different native languages.

Group Analytic Perspective

In the 1990s, there were huge socio-political changes and a war in our former country of Yugoslavia and our present country Serbia. The massive destruction was caused by violent behaviour of human beings who were at war. It led to terrible outcomes with catastrophic consequences. During and after this period, our patients brought their traumatic experiences to their individual and group therapies and we faced the impact those traumatic experiences had upon their internal end external lives, at the same time sharing the similar traumatizing context (Despotovic, 2002; Mojović, Despotovic and Satarić, 2014).

We were particularly interested in understanding the mourning processes in individuals and groups due to the traumatic experiences and losses (Despotovic and Satarić, 2011). Our psychotherapeutic work taught us that the mourning process was altered in groups and individuals. Myriad traumatic losses created a combination of internal, psychic space of the individual and the outer, social space. Outer and internal worlds became equated and devoid of good, loving objects. The confusion of boundaries between the inside and the outside was created (Kaës, 2019). The confusion was forced from the social space. The official media at that time persuaded the citizens that there was no war. The massive losses were powerful sources of schizo-paranoid and depressive anxieties and defences against them.

One of the main tasks of all individuals and the society as a whole in times of turmoil and disasters is to deal with traumatic losses and accept the reality of loss through the mourning process. It is the hypothesis of Millar (Millar, 2001) that traumatic losses make it just as hard for the groups, as for individuals, to tolerate mourning and to achieve a group identity that is tolerant to difference. He pointed out how serious and dangerous it could be when paranoid anxieties and "their extended defensive network when catastrophic loss of something good, somewhere known to have existed but which was destroyed…cannot be endured" (Millar, 2001).

It is worth mentioning that the group analysts and members of the therapy groups are permanently in contact with losses. It requires time and the whole group's endeavour to go through the "mourning work" (Freud, 1917), when each member terminates his/her therapy. The transient character of the therapy group membership does not diminish the value and beauty of learning through rich and meaningful relationships within the group despite the "revolt in the minds against mourning" (Freud, 1957) when an end comes. Mutual empathy may move the group and its members toward the reparation of a good internal object to test the reality of a loss. This painful but fruitful process moves the group toward maturity. The parts of the former members' identities stay as long as the group is alive, even when the therapy group membership is completely changed. They become part of the group culture, a legacy of accumulated historical group experience.

But mourning is uncertain in the presence of the members' traumatic experiences, which are usually cut off from the consciousness and verbal communication in the group. The breakdown of the symbolic functioning undermines the capacity for reflecting upon the lived experience. Painful thoughts and feelings are often impossible for the mind to hold, cannot be contained in memory as they are one of the most devastating consequences of trauma (Garland, 2018). Non-symbolized traumatic pieces of feelings and identities flow through the group matrix. The group is influenced by those cut off feelings through different actions that inhibit the group from mourning and developing deep and rich relationships.

It is obvious that the setting, the entity through which the therapist's container function was expressed, became even more important during last two decades of our work (Despotovic *et al.*, 2009). The setting had an active containing and holding function (Bion, 1959), which means to receive what the patient and the group communicate and to modify it into a form the group can integrate. It seemed essential to maintain this active container, not only to enable our patients to "gain access to the new relational world in which internal psychical reality becomes as real as external reality" (Quinodoz, 2018), but to differentiate what belonged to the internal reality of the individual or group from what belonged to the external reality. By keeping the setting alive, we stood on the borders of two overwhelming tendencies, from without and from within. Highly traumatic external reality intended to intrude the setting, massively attacking it, and our patients and groups expressed unconscious tendencies to threaten the setting (active container) as if it were container-as-a-thing.

An example of this is a shared fantasy that was verbalized in one therapy group: "When the bombing starts we will wait for the therapist in front of the Clinic." The members expressed a strong wish for external manifestation of the setting as a container, literally as a shelter or protective barrier against annihilation anxieties.

Some More Clinical Observations (Despotovic and Satarić, 2011):

- When a group member would experience an important loss, there was an absence of communication about the grief or it was very rare.
- Bringing the new member or sudden drop-out was followed by withdrawal or a depressed state of the mind of the group.
- Any changes were followed by regression to paranoid schizoid anxieties and primitive defences (denial, splitting, projective identification, omnipotence, manic defences, idealization, devaluation) and the group resistances in the form of scapegoating.
- Annihilation anxiety was deeply rooted in the group matrix.
- Regular breaks were followed by disproportional fear of disintegration of the therapy group and acting out (members were meeting outside the setting).
- As the conductors, we adopted a more active position with additional work to prevent a member with the traumatic loss to leave the therapy prematurely.
- Strong countertransference feelings, sometimes countertransference reactions (vivid memories 20 years later)
- Regular presence and staying in a state of reverie in spite of all uncertainties had been more effective than interpretations (Despotovic *et al.*, 2009)

An Example from Clinical Work

What follows is a presentation of the material from the slow open analytic group (therapist was TD) that started in 1998. The group met once a week for 90 minutes. It was heterogenous group, the members with traumatic experiences and losses were together with the members who needed therapy for other difficulties.

The wider social context was a very unstable socio-political situation. At the same day when the first session was held, the threat of the NATO bombing was abruptly announced. The bombing was cancelled, but for a while it was uncertain if the group could maintain its continuity. Membership fluctuated because some members emigrated suddenly and some moved temporarily due to the unsafe situation in the country, later coming back.

The members communicated their personal preoccupations and reasons for joining the therapy group, but from the beginning, the annihilation anxiety was rooted in the group matrix. One of the fantasies shared by the members of the group in a humorous way was that the group members could move their chairs to the part of the room away from the windows to avoid anticipated danger. It was interpreted as an illusion of being in the protected space in fear of danger.

During that period, there were few transference-countertransference actions. The most striking one was when one member came to the therapist in a panic to ask for written justification that could free him from joining the army in the conflict area and the therapist wrote it being aware of breaking a boundary.

A year later, when the NATO bombing really happened, the group sessions were cancelled, considering the complete uncertain external reality, and continued after a break of four months when the bombing ended. The wider social context at that moment was that the citizens massively protested against the government. Protests became part of our everyday life. The therapist acknowledged the importance of containing the annihilation anxieties by keeping a regular setting and never cancelled a single session. It reflected the need of the group to repair the initial disruptive period when the group was jeopardized even before it started.

The group survived. As the time was passing and the outer life stabilized after democratic changes in 2000, the group became mute of the past traumatic events end experiences.

Five years later, there were eight members, the majority of which had traumatic life experiences and traumatic losses. There were three more members who came for their therapy for different reasons, but their lives were not shattered by trauma and their voices at certain periods brought some stability for the group.

S was there from the start. He was suffering from "feeling nothing." He originated from nationally mixed marriage. When his parents divorced his father moved to another Republic where S loved to spend time during the summer with his step-mother and three new siblings. After the disintegration of Yugoslavia, he didn't see them for a decade. He denied any longing and called his father an "ultranationalist."

R, a young man, was a refugee who came to Serbia with his mother as a child from a region ravaged by war. His father stayed there, lost his leg in the war, but wanted to return in his home country. It resulted in his family being broken by the war. As a child, R was mistreated by the children because he spoke in a different dialect and he seriously fantasized about killing those children. He entered the group with an obsessive preoccupation that he was guilty of the death of his loving grandmother offering her a cup of coffee before she died.

M was a young woman, a nurse, and also a refugee as a child, who lived in a complete family that lost everything in the war with a seriously depressed mother. Her tormenting fear was that she would hurt an ill child while performing her duties as a nurse.

K was a young woman from a broken family with a violent father who accused her of the divorce of her parents and who cut her off. She had outbursts of rage.

V was the new member who entered the group after a few failures in her previous therapies. She was abandoned by her father and her mother was burdened by poverty in her childhood. Her family and brother who supported her financially lived in another state, which, during that period, became independent. V came for her University studies to Serbia but due to legislative changes, she lost her right to work legally but wanted to stay in Serbia. She was working endlessly on her graduation thesis about homeless people and struggled with existential issues.

When the new member was announced, R who wanted to end his therapy, remembered his aggressive fantasies toward his peers who mistreated him in school. He spoke about the weapons that all families owned in his birthplace and that everybody, even old women, knew how to shoot. *He retold his dream that he took the therapist to his birthplace.* Another member, M, also a refugee, with a mixture of shame and laughter said that then the therapist should know how to shoot. Other members, in a humorous, way wondered if they were in his dream imagining the therapist being there. It seemed a reminiscence of the "happy" childhood. But after a while, R remembered that his father lost his leg in the war and separated from his mother after the war, but still without pain. Only the therapist felt anxious, almost nauseous, but was later able to think about their fear of separation, an unconscious equation of the wounded father with the therapist and disruption by the change in the group after the new member came.

For the first time, some split off traumatic experiences were brought in and connected with relationships with the therapist and the group.

The group was again in a shaking period. What happened was that a terrible relationship was developed with the new member V. Unexpectedly, V was attacking everybody, was not ready to listen to others and was dismissing them for their "spoilt" lives. The group was trying to reach her, the three more mature members offered her different helpful ideas but in vain. After a while, half of the group members couldn't stand her. There were open quarrels without any resolution. The therapist's interventions that V was perceived as too different, or as an intruder, or mirror for others' fears were futile. We worked a lot on V's repetitive dream *that she was in dirty water like mud and trying unsuccessfully to get to clear water where other people swam, but there was an invisible line between, separating the two waters.*

The therapist understood that instead of noticing and overcoming the splitting in the group (within V too), the group fell into the "mud" of mixed but cut off feeling when exposed to V and her traumatic life full of losses and rage in relation to them. Just before the summer break, V suddenly lost her brother while not being aware that he was a substance addict. She left for her birthplace in another state. The therapist was in contact with her for a while, but V never came back and the group was frozen. For months, there was no way of opening the members' feelings about V dropping out, only the relief, which the therapist perceived as regressive absence of concern and loss of an inner empathic object. More mature members spoke with empathy that V was in their minds. Helplessness was seated in the therapist's countertransference for a while.

During that summer, S reunited with his family in another state and that revived some warm feelings in him. But there was another loss in the group. R lost his grandfather. He couldn't mourn and felt nothing but guilt and anxiety. After many group sessions, he accepted that he didn't kill his grandfather but became aware that he destroyed everything he achieved in his therapy because he felt as he did five years before, when he entered the group. He disturbed his parents, actually he made his father come from another state. He even slept with his mother and his father in the same bed, not being able to bear his anxiety. One member, with empathy, understood he finally reunited his parents, but another member K imagined a funny picture of him sleeping like a baby in the middle between his parents. Her laughter turned to sadness that her relationship with her father died. Sadness was felt in the whole group.

It is possible that R was sad about destroying his life and regressing his therapy to a child-like state for the sake of not letting go of his unfulfilled wish to have a complete family, that everybody was alive, healthy, living together at one place, maybe at his birthplace. Some members cried. The therapist went on to say that the group seemed like a complete, happy family when V was brought in the group. They hated listening to her unsolvable problems. They could feel like they lost the group and the therapist, and were furious at the therapist for destroying that "ideal" picture about us being together. R said he started to love the life he was living now…

We believe that the unconscious communications that contained pieces of feelings and experiences connected with traumatic experiences and losses needed to be worked through with the group as a whole. It seemed as if the group built an inflexible defensive structure that was used by the group to protect the members from going through traumatic experiences and enduring the pain of loss. It took many years of group struggle to reunite with those cut off pieces of identities that they "successfully" got rid of and placed somewhere: in another member, in the therapist or in the group as a whole. The group was saturated with rage. But the insight that the rage was part of the mourning process was missing. With so many traumatic experiences, the members were keeping alive the ideal objects (the broken families, broken childhood, the group). In such shattered worlds (internal and external), it was only to be expected. The more recent experiences with ending therapies in this group gave me some hope that it is possible to prevent trans-group, similar to trans-generational, transmission of the unmourned losses.

Discussion

During traumatization, the ego meets an overwhelming abundance of stimuli and impressions. The regulating functions of the mind breaks down and the processes of the psychic apparatus are pushed toward states of extreme anxiety and catastrophe (Rosenbaum and Varvin, 2007). Mental traces of such traumatic experiences are "wild" in the sense that the person has no capacity to organize and deal with them; no inner container in a relation to an inner empathic other that can help give meaning to experience (Laub, 2005). There is an experience of loss of internal protection — primarily the loss of the necessary feelings of basic trust and mastery. An empathic internal other is no longer functioning as a protective shield and the functions that give meaning to experiences may no longer work. Attachment to and trust in others may be perceived as dangerous, a reminder of previous catastrophes. Relating to others, for example a psychoanalyst, may be felt as a risk of re-experiencing the original helplessness and a feeling of being left alone in utter despair. The traumatized patient will from the start of therapy involve the analyst in a not symbolized and unconscious relationship where the patient communicates by acting out and in this way presents important aspects of their traumatic experiences (S Varvin, 2013). Withdrawal patterns may be the consequence, creating a negative spiral as withdrawal at the same time means the loss of potential external support (Varvin and Rosenbaum, 2018). Traumatization may thus affect several dimensions of the person's relations with the external world and give disturbances on the bodily-affective level, on the capacity to form relations to others and the group and family and on the ability to give meaning to experience. The last is dependent on the social and cultural meaning-giving functions that, under normal circumstances, provide affirmative narratives (e.g., stories told by elders), scientific explanations (e.g., psychological theories) and political acknowledgement (e.g., leaders' acknowledging the historical circumstances of the atrocity).

Massive traumatization creates destabilization of the basic structures of human relationships on the level of intimate relationships where intrapsychic and interpersonal functions concern regulations of emotions, primary care functions and basic identity issues; on the level of the individual relations to the group where personal identity and developmental task are negotiated; and on the cultural or discourse level, where narratives are established that give meaning to and stabilize relations and developments on the individual and group levels (Rosenbaum and Varvin, 2007; Rosenbaum, Jovic and Varvin, 2020). Any approach to patients who have been traumatized in a violent social context, such as wars, mass persecution and genocide, must therefore be sensitive to, and take into consideration the dimensions of social and cultural influences on development, psychopathology and health-sickness behaviour.

An enactment involves a collapse in the therapeutic dialogue where the analyst is drawn into an interaction where she/he unwittingly acts, thereby actualizing unconscious wishes of both him/her-self and the patient. It may be a definable episode in a process with more or less clear distinctions between the pre-phase, the actual moment and the post-phase, but may also be part of a prolonged process in therapy (Jacobs, 1986). Enactment appears, thus, as an unintentional breakdown of the analytic rule of "speech not act," and this may imply a new opportunity of integration or it may hinder the analytic process when it goes unnoticed or unanalyzed. What the patient communicates touches the analyst and may hook on to the unconscious, not worked through material on his/her side, resulting in an action that, at first sight, is not therapeutic, therefore named countertransference enactment (Jacobs, 1986). Such enactments on the analyst side may, however, be a starting point for a possible process of symbolization and becoming conscious of these implicit experiences. Enactments may represent the possibility for symbolizing material related to traumatic experiences and lay the groundwork for remembering, not only "recalling" or "evoking." It implies the transmutation of some material into a new form in order to be brought into the psychic field where the functions of remembering and integration can occur (Scarfone, 2011). Enactments can, thus, in this context, be seen as the actualization of relational scripts or scenarios where unconscious, not-symbolized material is activated both in the patient and in the analyst. This is seen as an unavoidable part of the analytic interaction and the outcome depends on the analytic couple's ability to bring the enactment into the psychic field.

Lack of social support and recognition has for many traumatized persons been devastating. Treatment of traumatized patients can therefore only with great difficulties work in a social/cultural setting where traumatization is not acknowledged or worked with at other levels in society. Patients with complex trauma often live in difficult social, economic, and cultural situations Treatment and rehabilitation need, therefore, to be conducted often by a team and when and how to implement psychoanalytic therapy, must be carefully evaluated and will need constant support from the team and other social services.

Conclusion

We have in this chapter argued for psychoanalytic understanding of extreme traumatization and its consequences and for psychoanalytic psychotherapy as a treatment that represents a holistic approach that can relate to traumatized persons' and groups' complex problems. We hold that any approach to patients who have been traumatized in a violent social context, must be sensitive to, and take into consideration the dimensions of social and cultural influences on development, psychopathology, and health-sickness behaviour. Extreme traumatization may have profound effects on basic mental functioning and on the function of groups and societies. The aim of therapy must be to help the patient create a more secure inner psychic reality and to be more able to function and create trust in the external reality. Psychotherapy is therefore thoroughly dependent on society's acceptance of the traumatizing reality, of traumatized persons and of social support and help integration.

A narrow focus on a psychiatrically defined diagnosis such as PTSD, will therefore be insufficient for most, even if these more trauma-focused therapies may give some help. We can say that the posttraumatic symptomatology presented in a form of PTSD can be understood as an initiation of posttraumatic process, but that the more complex and damaging might be a chronic and silent manifestation that we can probably understand only in a psychoanalytical treatment — either in individual or group psychotherapy. In that sense, the main aim of therapy and the therapist is to unlock the mourning process, support it within the psychoanalytical setting and work in a transference/countertransference relationship. We see the psychoanalytic approaches described in this chapter (individual and group therapy) as basically re-humanizing approaches for human beings who have been through human-made hell on earth.

Under normal circumstances, becoming a human goes through a long development process of caretaking, trust building and learning to be a member of a group/society while at the same time being a unique, independent individual. Extreme traumatization aims at destroying what has been built all through a person's life. For many, the rebuilding of trust and mental capacities may take a long time, even the rest of the person's life. Psychoanalytic therapy offers a way to start this process through its stability and constant focus on the humanness of our existence.

References

Acarturk, C. *et al.* (2015) 'EMDR for Syrian refugees with posttraumatic stress disorder symptoms: Results of a pilot randomized controlled trial', *European Journal of Psychotraumatology*, 6(1), p. 27414.

American Psychiatric Association (1980) *Diagnostic and Statistical Manual of Mental Disorders, 3rd Edition*. Washington, DC: American Psychiatric Association.

Betancourt, T. S. *et al.* (2015) 'We left one war and came to another: Resource loss, acculturative stress, and caregiver–child relationships in Somali refugee families', *Cultural Diversity and Ethnic Minority Psychology*, 21(1), p. 114.

Bion, W. (1977) *Seven Servants*. New York: Aronson.

Bion, W. R. (1959) *Experiences in Groups*. London & New York: Routledge.

Bogic, M., Njoku, A. and Priebe, S. (2015) 'Long-term mental health of war-refugees: a systematic literature review', *BMC International Health and Human Rights*, 15(1), p. 29. doi: 10.1186/s12914-015-0064-9.

Despotovic, T. (2002) 'Functioning of Institutions and Helplessness - The Evolution of Emotional Reaction of Helpers', in *Help the Helpers*. Belgrade: Save the Children, UK, pp. 50–56.

Despotovic, T. *et al.* (2009) 'Positive and Negative Containment of Social Fragmentation Mirrored in Group Analytic Process, in Prague: presented at EFPP Group Section Conference.

Despotovic, T. and Satarić, J. (2011) 'Loss Definite, Mourning Uncertain', in *15th European Group Analytic Symposium*. London: GASI Symposium.

Fazel, M. *et al.* (2012) 'Mental health of displaced and refugee children resettled in high-income countries: risk and protective factors', *The Lancet*, 379(9812), pp. 266–282.

Fazel, M., Wheeler, J. and Danesh, J. (2005) 'Prevalence of serious mental disorder in 7000 refugees resettled in western countries: a systematic review', *The Lancet*, 365(9467), pp. 1309–1314. doi: https://doi.org/10.1016/S0140-6736(05)61027-6.

Follette, W. C. and Houts, A. C. (1996) 'Models of scientific progress and the role of theory in taxonomy development: A case study of the DSM', *Journal of Consulting and Clinical Psychology*, 64(6), p. 1120.

Freedman, N. *et al.* (2018) *Another Kind of Evidence: Studies on Internalization, Annihilation Anxiety, and Progressive Symbolization in the Psychoanalytic Process*. Routledge.

Freud, S. (1917) 'Mourning and melancholia', in *The Standard Edition of the Complete Psychological Works of Sigmund Freud, Volume XIV (1914-1916): On the History of the Psycho-Analytic Movement, Papers on Metapsychology and Other Works*, pp. 237–258.

Freud, S. (1957) 'On transience', in *The Standard Edition of the Complete Psychological Works of Sigmund Freud, Volume XIV (1914-1916): On the History of the Psycho-Analytic Movement, Papers on Metapsychology and Other Works*, pp. 303–307.

Gammeltoft-Hansen, T. (2016) *Hvordan løser vi flygtningekrisen?* Informations forlag.

Garland, C. (2018) 'The traumatised group', in *Understanding trauma*. Routledge, pp. 183–198.

Hassan, G. *et al.* (2016) 'Mental health and psychosocial wellbeing of Syrians affected by armed conflict', *Epidemiology and Psychiatric Sciences*, 25(2), pp. 129–141.

Hocking, D. C., Kennedy, G. A. and Sundram, S. (2015) 'Mental disorders in asylum seekers: The role of the refugee determination process and employment', *The Journal of Nervous and Mental Disease*, 203(1), pp. 28–32.

Hurvich, M. (2003) 'The place of annihilation anxieties in psychoanalytic theory', *Journal of The American Psychoanalytic Association*, 51(2), pp. 579–616.

Hurvich, M. (2015) 'Vernichtungsängste-traumatische Ängste', *Psyche*, 69(9–10), pp. 797–825.

Jacobs, T. J. (1986) 'On countertransference enactments', *Journal of the American Psychoanalytic Association*, 34(2), pp. 289–307.
Jović, V. (2018) 'Working with Traumatized Refugees on the Balkan Route', *International Journal of Applied Psychoanalytic Studies*. pp. 187 –201.
Kaës, R. (2019) *L'institution et les institutions: études psychanalytiques*. Dunod.
Lacan, J. (1977) *Écrits*. Hammondsworth: Penguin Books.
Laub, D. (2005) 'Traumatic shutdown of narrative and symbolization: A death instinct derivative?', *Contemporary Psychoanalysis*, 41(2), pp. 307–326.
Laub, D. and Podell, D. (1995) 'Art and trauma', *International Journal of Psycho-Analysis*, 76, pp. 991–1005.
Lecours, S. and Bouchard, M.-A. (1997) 'Dimensions of mentalisation: Outlining levels of psychic transformation', *The International Journal of Psycho-analysis*, 78(5), p. 855.
Leuzinger-Bohleber, M. (2012) Changes in dreams—From a psychoanalysis with a traumatised, chronic depressed patient. London: Karnac Books.
Mayes, R. and Horwitz, A. V. (2005) 'DSM-III and the revolution in the classification of mental illness', *Journal of the History of the Behavioral Sciences*, 41(3), pp. 249–267.
Millar, D. (2001) 'A psychoanalytic view of biblical myth 1', *The International Journal of Psychoanalysis*, 82(5), pp. 965–979.
Mojović, M., Despotovic, T. and Satarić, J. (2014) "Conception Trauma' of Group Analysis in Serbia', *Group Analysis*, 47(2), pp. 113–127.
Nickerson, A. *et al.* (2014) 'Posttraumatic stress disorder and prolonged grief in refugees exposed to trauma and loss', *BMC psychiatry*, 14(1), pp. 1–11.
Opaas, M. and Varvin, S. (2015) 'Relationships of childhood adverse experiences with mental health and quality of life at treatment start for adult refugees traumatized by pre-flight experiences of war and human rights violations', *The Journal of Nervous and Mental Disease*, 203(9), p. 684.
Opaas, M., Wentzel-Larsen, T. and Varvin, S. (2020) 'The 10-year course of mental health, quality of life, and exile life functioning in traumatized refugees from treatment start', *Plos One*, 15(12), p. e0244730.
Priebe, S. *et al.* (2010) 'Experience of human rights violations and subsequent mental disorders–A study following the war in the Balkans', *Social Science & Medicine*, 71(12), pp. 2170–2177.
PTSD Treatment Basics - PTSD: National Center for PTSD (no date). Available at: https://www.ptsd.va.gov/understand_tx/tx_basics.asp (Accessed: 29 December 2019).
Purnell, C. (2010) 'Childhood trauma and adult attachment', *Healthcare Counselling and Psychotherapy Journal*, 10(2), pp. 1–7.
Quinodoz, J.-M. (2018) 'Teaching Freud's "Mourning and Melancholia"', in On Freud's. Routledge, pp. 179–192.
Rosenbaum, B., Jovic, V. and Varvin, S. (2020) 'Understanding the refugee-traumatised persons', *Psychosozial*, 43(3), pp. 11–23. doi: 10.30820/0171-3434-2020-3-11
Rosenbaum, B. and Varvin, S. (2007) 'The influence of extreme traumatization on body, mind and social relations', *The International Journal of Psychoanalysis*, 88(6), pp. 1527–1542. doi: 10.1111/j.1745-8315.2007.tb00758.x
Sabes-Figuera, R. *et al.* (2012) 'Long-term impact of war on healthcare costs: An eight-country study', *PloS One*, 7(1), p. e29603.

Sagbakken, M., Bregård, I. M. and Varvin, S. (2020) 'The past, the present, and the future: A qualitative study exploring how refugees' experience of time influences their mental health and well-being', *Frontiers in Sociology*, p. 46. Available at: https://www.frontiersin.org/article/10.3389/fsoc.2020.00046.

Scarfone, D. (2011) 'Repetition: Between presence and meaning', *Canadian Journal of Psychoanalysis*, 19(1), pp. 70–86.

Schottenbauer, M. A. *et al.* (2008) 'Nonresponse and dropout rates in outcome studies on PTSD: Review and methodological considerations', *Psychiatry: Interpersonal and Biological Processes*, 71(2), pp. 134–168.

Shatan, C. F. (1972) *Post-Vietnam Syndrome, The New York Times*. Available at: http://www.nytimes.com/1972/05/06/archives/postvietnam-syndrome.html (Accessed: 8 February 2018).

Shephard, B. (2001) *The War on Nerves: Soldiers and Psychiatrists in the Twentieth Century*. Cambridge Massachusetts: Harvard University Press.

Sleijpen, M. *et al.* (2016) 'Between power and powerlessness: a meta-ethnography of sources of resilience in young refugees', *Ethnicity & Health*, 21(2), pp. 158–180.

Taft, C. T. *et al.* (2007) 'Posttraumatic stress disorder symptoms, physiological reactivity, alcohol problems, and aggression among military veterans.' *Journal of Abnormal Psychology*, 116(3), p. 498.

Ungar, M. (2012) *The Social Ecology of resilience. A Handbook of Theory and Practice*. New York, Dordrecht, Heidelberg, London: Springer Verlag.

UNHCR (2016) *Regional Refugee & Resilience Plan 2015-2016. In response to the Syria crisis*. Available at: https://www.unhcr.org/54918efa9.html (Accessed: 20 September 2021).

Vaage, A. B. *et al.* (2010) 'Long-term mental health of Vietnamese refugees in the aftermath of trauma', *The British Journal of Psychiatry*, 196(2), pp. 122–125.

Van der Kolk, B. A. (1994) 'The body keeps the score: Memory and the evolving psychobiology of posttraumatic stress', *Harvard Review of Psychiatry*, 1(5), pp. 253–265.

Van der Kolk, B. A. and McFarlane, A. C. (1996) *Traumatic Stress: The Effects of Overwhelming Experience on Mind, Body, and Society*. Guilford Press.

Varvin, S (2013) 'Trauma als Nonverbaler Kommunikation', *Zeitschrift für psychoanalytische Theorie und Praxis*, 28, pp. 114–130.

Varvin, S. (2003) *Mental Survival Strategies after Extreme Traumatisation*. Copenhagen: Multivers.

Varvin, S. (2015) 'Trauma and resilience', *Psychoanalysis, Collective Traumas and Memory Places*, 4, p. 191.

Varvin, S. (2016) 'Psychoanalysis with the traumatized patient: Helping to survive extreme experiences and complicated loss', in *International Forum of Psychoanalysis*. Taylor & Francis, pp. 73–80.

Varvin, S. (2017) 'Our relations to refugees: Between compassion and dehumanization', *The American Journal of Psychoanalysis*, 77(4), pp. 359–377. doi: 10.1057/s11231-017-9119-0.

Varvin, Sverre (2013) 'Psychoanalyse mit Traumatisierten', in *Forum der Psychoanalyse*. Springer, pp. 373–389.

Varvin, S. and Rosenbaum, B. (2018) 'Severely traumatized patients' attempts at reorganizing their relations to others in psychotherapy: An enunciation analysis', in *Another Kind of Evidence*. Routledge, pp. 167–182.

Varvin, S. and Stiles, W. (1999) 'Emergence of severe traumatic experiences: An assimilation analysis of psychoanalytic therapy with a political refugee', *Psychotherapy Research*, 9(3), pp. 381–404.

Vitriol, V. G. *et al.* (2009) 'Evaluation of an outpatient intervention for women with severe depression and a history of childhood trauma', *Psychiatric services*, 60(7), pp. 936–942.

Weber, B. (2017) *The EU-Turkey Refugee Deal and the Not Quite Closed Balkan Route*. Sarajevo. Available at: http://library.fes.de/pdf-files/bueros/sarajevo/13436.pdf.

Wong, E. C. *et al.* (2015) 'Characterizing the mental health care of US Cambodian refugees', *Psychiatric Services*, 66(9), pp. 980–984.

Young, A. (1995) *The Harmony of Illusions: Inventing Post-traumatic Stress Disorder*. Princeton, NJ: Princeton University Press.

Chapter 14

The Impact of Social Trauma on Group Analytic Theory

Morris Nitsun

Introduction

We live in an age of trauma. An air of traumatic uncertainty or feared trauma in the wider world as well as trauma in individual lives, often through violence or abuse, is increasingly uncovered and exposed. Not surprisingly, we as psychologists and psychotherapists are paying considerable attention to trauma. There are now many models of trauma and its consequences. It has, in recent years, become a prominent theme in group analytic literature. For example, much of the current work on the social unconscious (Hopper and Weinberg 2011) emphasizes trauma as a core contributor to the social unconscious, often leading to the dissociation and denial of experience that feeds the unconscious but that may be transmitted unprocessed down the generational line. In my own work on the Anti-group (Nitsun 1996, 2015), I have given trauma an important place in generating the anxiety and aversion to group participation that can lead to group division and disintegration. Although many of us have taken trauma as a subject, what we have not looked at is how trauma may have affected us personally and what influence this has had on our writing, both as individual authors and as a collective voice in the development of theory: how trauma impacts our theoretical beliefs. We know that writers select what they write about for a variety of reasons, that their chosen themes not uncommonly relate to themselves, whether directly or indirectly, and that their own personal histories may influence the subjects to which they give their greatest attention. We also know intuitively that many of us are attracted to group analysis because we are struggling with issues of identity and belonging, perhaps hoping that becoming group analysts will help not just our patients, but ourselves, to find a home. I suggest we may also be attracted to the field because we live in the shadow of trauma, since most families and individual lives are affected in some way by trauma, and there is the hope that our theory and practice, including the models we have created ourselves, will help us to get to grapple with the shadows of the past.

DOI: 10.4324/9781003269649-20

In this chapter, I aim to look at the impact of trauma on the development of group analysis. My main focus is on Foulkes as the founder of group analysis, but I will explore the history of Northfield hospital in the mid-20th century, and I will also refer to Freud and his reaction to trauma as a contrasting example to Foulkes. Much of this revolves around World War II and the reactions of these eminent figures to the war. I also later in the chapter refer to my own experience of growing up in South Africa during the apartheid years, my family's Holocaust background and the effect that had on my development as a group analyst and a writer in the field. I want in this chapter to adopt an approach that considers both the distorting and restrictive influence of trauma and its generative challenge: the destructive and the creative and the dialectic that links the two. We are generally, and not surprisingly, more familiar with a negative view of trauma and its consequences. We know about the adverse consequences in people's lives, the painful symptoms of depression, dissociation and depersonalization, as well as the marked interpersonal and social dysfunction that are the result of trauma. We know that trauma usually induces a sense of helplessness and loss of control, that it distorts memory and imagination and that it can have a paralyzing effect on development. I will come back to this later in this chapter, since the destructive effects of trauma cannot and must not be avoided, but what I want to highlight here is the idea that trauma can have a creative influence. We can see this in two ways. The experience of trauma generates a wish to put things right, to repair, to support the healing process. This is usually where our treatments take place, to help people survive the impasse of trauma and move beyond it. There is a growing literature supporting this idea of post-traumatic growth, some of it presented by Calhoun and Tedeschi (2014) in their "Handbook of Posttraumatic Growth." But there is another sense in which trauma may have a creative impact: at a broader, existential level. We seek to overcome life's arbitrary and often cruel impingements—the "slings and arrows of outrageous fortune," in Shakespeare's words—and instead become agents of change and not just victims. We seek to transcend the trauma and this may be a source of great creativity.

Northfield

I want to begin with Northfield Hospital in the 1940s and the so-called Northfield experiments that have a crucial place in the history of group analysis. Most British people will be aware of this because it is a part of British history. But for those who don't know, Northfield Hospital was a military hospital near the city of Birmingham that became a center for treating many soldiers returning "shell-shocked," to use an old-fashioned term for traumatized, from the World War II. The hospital attracted many eminent clinicians to work there, including key figures like Sigmund H. Foulkes,

Wilfred. R. Bion, Harold Bridger and Tom Main, all of whom contributed to a significant spurt in the development of mental health treatment, groupwork in particular.

The Northfield experiments refer to two highly productive periods in which first Bion and later Foulkes initiated treatment programs in the hospital. These two had different approaches and it seems that Foulkes was more successful than Bion in winning the trust of the military leadership and remaining in a leadership capacity for much longer. But whatever the differences between Bion and Foulkes, and there certainly were differences that later became institutionalized splits, there also were important similarities. Both strove to inculcate a democratic culture in the hospital and to encourage the men to take responsibility not just for themselves but also for their fellow soldiers and their community. The methods used were very much group methods, ranging from group occupational and recreational activities to regular discussion groups in which the men were encouraged to talk about themselves and their concerns. These were like group therapy even if not called as such. There are reports of how this drab provincial hospital, particularly under Foulkes, became a lively center, bursting with activity and creativity. Importantly for us, it was the forerunner of therapeutic communities, it stimulated the widespread application of group psychotherapy in the United Kingdom (UK) and it provided opportunities for the early organizational application of group methods. It was arguably *the* creative moment in the evolution of group methods in Britain from which spread further developments through Europe. This is reflected in the 2018 EFPP Conference in Belgrade, which has attracted a large number of Europeans many of whom have inherited the creative legacy of Foulkes, Bion and other figures in the group field.

Northfield and its innovations would not have happened had it not been for World War II. The experiments were in large part a response to the dramatically increased need for treating soldiers returning with battle fatigue and many associated illnesses. The group approach was advantageous: all these men could simply not have been reached with individual psychotherapy. Group methods were clearly the way forward. But as Tom Harrison (2000) points out in his book "Bion, Rickman, Foulkes and the Northfield Experiments," it was not just a response to clinical need. It was also the vision of people like Bion and Foulkes, their growing interest in groups and their courage to experiment, that enabled these developments to take place. It was a moment of creative fusion: many talents, skills and strengths coming together in a powerful synergy that fired the entire group movement in the UK and later parts of Europe. This is an example of how trauma on the scale of a world war generated a highly creative process that influenced theory and practice for generations to come.

Foulkes

I want now to take a closer look at Foulkes in terms of his own history and theory development and what we may imagine was his personal trauma during the war, having left Nazi Germany and immigrated to the UK in 1933. By the time of his death in 1976, Foulkes had made a highly creative contribution: starting group analysis in the UK, building his theory and actively applying group methods in the services he led as a psychiatrist in the British National Health Service (NHS). He was also a teacher and inspired many of students to train further in group methods. What emerged was a very positive, optimistic account of the healing potential of groups (Foulkes 1948, 1964). Some of the concepts Foulkes formulated, such as the group matrix, mirroring and resonance, remain the cornerstone of group analysis and, while he grappled with the more complex processes that occur in groups, Foulkes never lost sight of the fundamental power of people openly talking to each other. In this way, the energy of ordinary human conversations could be harnessed and transformed into something extraordinary in people's development.

The problem, as I pointed out in my 1996 book on the Anti-group, was that, as I saw it, Foulkes neglected the darker side of groups, not just the aggression and hostility that can arise in the group, but the overall ambivalence people may have to groups, sometimes amounting to great suspicion and hostility and a marked fear of becoming part of a group. When I trained as a group analyst, I was the head of a large psychology department in the NHS and was setting out to establish a comprehensive program of therapy groups. This is one of the reasons I did the training: to equip myself with the knowledge and skills I needed to head this service. But what I discovered was a considerable gap between the theory of group analysis and the practice. There simply were far more problems than could be accounted for in group analytic terms, in particular the fall-out from groups, the potentially high drop-out rate, the dissatisfaction with the group approach, the conflicts and difficulties in groups that could not be resolved and sometimes the diminution and even disintegration of groups. Additionally, I found there was organizational resistance to groups. My main hospital base at the time was suspicious of groups and not infrequently groups were sabotaged, usually unthinkingly, but nevertheless making it very difficult to develop a robust group culture. In the end, I did succeed in building a strong group program, but it was not without a struggle and the patience and dedication of the staff working with me.

The reason I am sharing this is that I want to highlight the significant gaps in the theory. It seemed to me that the group analytic community at the time had an idealized view of groups, that Foulkes gave a sometimes idealized account of groups and that he in turn was idealized by his increasing number of followers. I have to explain myself here. I have sometimes been accused of adopting too critical a perspective of Foulkes. A group analytic colleague once said to me that I had a prejudiced view: that it all depends on how one reads Foulkes and that he, my colleague, did not see the idealization in the way I did. I take the point, recognizing that we indeed bring our own beliefs and biases to the table, but I like to think of myself as a fair judge based on long-standing experience as a psychologist and psychotherapist and I wanted my concerns to be taken seriously.

I have previously raised the question of what—assuming I am right—it was that led Foulkes to present a largely one-sided view of groups. And this is where I come back to my theme of trauma. Foulkes himself did not escape the horrors of World War II. According to reports, he lost at least one member to the Nazi onslaught and some reports say that he lost half his family. He also had to leave Germany as a refugee and start a new life in England. We do not have enough information about Foulkes to know whether this actually constituted a trauma for him — and this is another significant feature of Foulkes, that there is surprisingly little biographical material to help us to understand exactly what these experiences meant to him. Foulkes himself wrote very little about his war experiences and that of immigration. However, it is hard not to conclude that there must have some element at least of trauma. It is the lack of clarity about this, about this vital part of Foulkes' life, that leads me to propose a gap. Not unusually in post-traumatic stress reactions there is a gap: a gap in continuity, as if an aspect of experience had been blanked off. If this is true in Foulkes' case, it suggests a link between Foulkes' neglect of group aggression and his own difficulty in processing and assimilating his experience during and perhaps following the war. Whereas I see his participation at Northfield as part of a creative attempt to deal with the war and its aftermath, I see the gaps in his theory as the product of dissociation or denial of "the facts of reality." How else, while World War II was raging, while human groups were behaving in the most barbaric ways imaginable, while he himself had been a victim of the violence of war, could Foulkes have written such a positive account of groups? The point I am making is about the disfiguring effects of trauma that linger through the operation of defenses, such as dissociation and denial, however badly needed these defenses are in order to survive. Or, and still in line with my hypothesis, was Foulkes' determination to evolve a positive and generative group culture in his writing on group psychotherapy also a creative gesture: a form of reparation, of making good the damage of the past, a hope perhaps of creating not just better groups but a better world?

Some of you will know that Foulkes changed his name several times. Starting life as German-Jewish Siegmund Heinrich Fuchs, he changed his name in England to S. H. Foulkes and later was known as very English Michael Foulkes. There have been various interpretations of these name changes. There were probably practical reasons for the changes, including the tendency of Jews living in England at the time of World War II to Anglicize their names, probably as a protective device. But each time Foulkes did this, was he disowning or dissociating some aspect of his identity and his past (Bledin 2004)?

Freud

I would like briefly to bring in Sigmund Freud in terms of Freud's response to the war at the time he emigrated to England in 1938. Freud, who also lost half his family in the Holocaust and who emigrated to England in circumstances of great fear, with the Nazis in close pursuit, wrote his most far-reachingly pessimistic work in the last phase of his life. His theory of the death instinct and the self-destructive nature of human beings was a product of this time, already reflected in his book "Civilisation and its Discontents," published in 1930 and considered a response to the experience of the first World War. His last book, "Analysis Terminable and Interminable," published in 1937, was focused more on psychoanalytic treatment and his doubts about treatment outcomes, questioningly very openly widespread assumptions about cure. The writer Thompson (1991) has highlighted Freud's courage in questioning in his last years the validity of his life's work. A distinct vein of pessimism had crept into his writing, but Thompson regards this as "corrective pessimism." Freud's aim was not to eradicate psychoanalysis but to restore therapeutic balance, to highlight the importance of impasse and failure in analytic treatment. This can be compared with Foulkes whose writing on groups at a very similar time had the clarion call of optimism and, as I saw it, little consideration of the risks, problems and limitations of group analytic treatment.

There were important differences between the two men, of course. Freud when he came to England, was much older, chronically ill with cancer and nearing the end of his life. Foulkes was a young man, about 37, in good health, with most of his life ahead of him and the challenge of re-establishing himself professionally and personally in a new country. Also, Freud was reviewing his work at a very late stage of life, whereas Foulkes had embarked on a new project of great promise and potential. Could these differences account for their different psychoanalytic perspectives, for the very different tone of their writing and for their contribution to theory? Or did these represent two different ways of relating to personal and social trauma? Also, how much does stage of life and current experience determine what occupies us most and infiltrates our writing?

Interestingly, Foulkes met Freud on only one occasion in his life. This was in 1936 when Foulkes went to visit Freud in Vienna. This was a significant meeting as Foulkes was profoundly influenced by Freud and remained so throughout his life, even when his model shifted more and more toward group analysis. Foulkes describes the meeting in a paper published in 1969 in response to a request from The Sigmund Freud Archives in New York and published in "Selected Papers" in 1990. Perhaps the most striking moment in Foulkes' account is when Freud asked Foulkes how old he was. When Foulkes replied that he was 38, Freud commented "What terrible things you may have yet to experience." Of course, Freud was right and Foulkes acknowledges this in the paper. Freud's words were prophetic because Foulkes saw the eruption of war and its consequences. He must have known all about trauma and social destruction. Yet he chose a reparative and creative path, for which we owe him a debt of gratitude, at the same time, as I see it, neglecting to incorporate in his theory the weight of conflict and aggression that was and is a reality of so many lives.

Myself

In the last part of this chapter, I want to bring myself in, in terms of my experience of growing up in South Africa, the child of Jewish parents with a history of persecution. I have to acknowledge that when it comes to trauma as a lived experience, I was more fortunate than either Freud or Foulkes. I was never directly affected by war. When I left South Africa to live in the UK, it was a personal choice, not a response to immediate threat. However, my upbringing was in the shadow of a violent South African history and the dawning reality of the Holocaust that had just happened in Europe (I was born in 1943) and that had affected my family.

As far as apartheid is concerned, I was of course in the privileged minority group of Whites. But growing up in a small rural town in the Cape Province of South Africa, I was keenly aware of the enforced divisions between people, the suffering this produced, and later as I grew into adulthood, the secrecy and violence with which the government set about implementing the doctrine of apartheid. As one of the very few Jewish families in a small Afrikaans town, I was aware of the threat of isolation and humiliation, the fear that we could be targeted as the next despised group. I grew up in a very anxious, divided society. I believe everyone was tainted by apartheid, not just those who were black.

Additionally, there was the history of my parents' families. My mother's family was for some years exiled from Lithuania to Siberia on the pretext of their being spies; they lived there in dire poverty, losing at least one child to starvation. Interestingly, my mother did speak about this, recalling the hunger and the way the family struggled to survive. My father, by contrast, never spoke about his family's Holocaust background, even though we knew the broad facts. He had emigrated to South Africa in the 1920s leaving behind, also in Lithuania, half his family, all of whom were killed at roughly the time that I was born. After World War II, there was a prevailing silence on the Holocaust in South Africa. The first I got to know of it was when as an early adolescent I came across photographs of concentration camp life in a book on Jewish history. There were pictures of emaciated victims, of the death trains, of people being herded and executed in groups, of piles of shoes, of teeth and eyeglasses. I was shocked and yet, sensing the deep shame in my family, I said nothing. Only later, many years later, did I take it upon myself to ask my father what had happened. He was very taken aback by my question, a question it seems no one had dared ask him, and I noticed this proud man, my father, shrinking under the weight of the question. He then did tell me all that he knew. But it was not a complete story. He did not know exactly what happened to his family in the end. Their letters from abroad, having previously come quite regularly, had stopped abruptly but he did not know why and he had not been able to find out how they met their death. Of course, if this were today with the benefit of the Internet, it would have been much easier to find out. But my father might still have wanted to avoid the facts, since the Jews in Lithuania were treated in a particularly violent and brutal way. Perhaps this saved him more pain but at the expense of the great sadness and anxiety that increasingly became a feature of my family.

Why am I sharing this? It may be that I myself need to share it in a setting on social trauma where I can talk freely about it. But more than that, I have to consider that it was these experiences in South Africa, against the background of World War II in Europe, that made me acutely aware of what, for me, was missing in the group analytic literature — the fundamental fact of how groups may be prone to aggression and how the larger the scale of the group, how much more intense the aggression could become. Of course, Foulkes was writing about psychotherapy, not war, and understandably he wanted to convey the collaborative potential of groups. But even then, therapy groups very much had to deal with aggressive and destructive fantasies and impulses. Without a framework within which we can understand this, we may be less than qualified and able to deal with it. This is why I introduced the notion of the Anti-group in publications in the 1990s and more recently in a 2015 book. Without realizing it at the time, I believe I was attempting to bridge the gaps in my own family history, to fill the breach created by dissociation and denial. Interestingly, there were some hostile reactions to my first book, which left me with the feeling that my observations were seen as an act of disloyalty and aggression, of taking a position that was unfairly challenging, of over-emphasizing a particular point. Perhaps they were right, if indeed I was coming so much from personal history.

Further developments in the family....

The issue of the Holocaust was never discussed again in my family; it went with my father to his grave.

The impact on successive generations: the psychotic boy, my nephew, who broke down following a motor accident in which his best friend was killed and another friend seriously injured. My nephew survived physically but almost immediately had a psychotic lapse from which he has not recovered. His psychosis was attributed to over-use of drugs but, as far as I could see, no one discussed in any depth the impact of the fatal accident.

I wondered whether this reflected transmission through the generations of my father's social trauma and loss — that was not openly discussed or processed.

Conclusion

I want to end with some comments about the social unconscious and how as writers, we ourselves relate to it, embody it, represent it or may even collude with it. The concept of the social unconscious has become prominent in much of the recent writing on group analysis, the emphasis being on the power of the silent, the unsaid, the repressed aspects of society and culture to affect us in significant and sometimes detrimental ways. Although the concept had its origins in the writing of other authors, such as Erich Fromm, it was Foulkes who brought it to light within the group analytic context. He did not develop it in much detail, but it was subsequently taken up and expanded greatly by other group analysts. It is ironic that it was Foulkes who introduced the concept, given what I believe was his own difficulty in acknowledging the facts of history as they affected him and his family. Perhaps he was intuitively aware of the gap in his consciousness – or at least the aspects that he was unable to share in his writing. Hence, he highlighted the concept, while himself struggling with the very process, paradoxically concealing the lived experiences and the problems of communication that informed his contribution to the social unconscious. But perhaps this is how theory develops over the longer term. No one theorist can say it all. We are all products of the time we grew up in, with our blind spots and limitations. Additionally, the world we live in changes contextually and culturally all the time and what pertains to one period of time may not to another. Theory is of necessity revisited and revised. But I want to conclude on the idea that our theories, to some extent at least, may emerge from a matrix of trauma. Some of the greatest works of literature, both within and outside the psychotherapies, have their origins in the experience of trauma and the different ways each of us finds to face trauma and survive. I hope I have shown that this may have both creative and restrictive aspects. I have concentrated on Foulkes and the origins of group analysis in this chapter but the impact of social trauma, which is at the same time always personal trauma, on the development of theory may be a fruitful path to pursue more generally in the evolution of the psychotherapies.

References

Bledin, K (2004) What's in a name? Foulkes, identity and the social unconscious. Group Analysis, 37, 475–487

Calhoun, LG and Tedeschi, RG (2014) A Handbook of Post-Traumatic Growth. London: Psychology Press

Foulkes, E (ed) (1990) Selected Papers of SH Foulkes. London: Karnac

Foulkes, SH (1948) Introduction to Group Analytic Psychotherapy. London: Heinemann

Foulkes, SH (1964) Therapeutic Group Analysis. London: Allen and Unwin

Harrison, T (2000) Bion, Rickman, Foulkes and the Northfield Experiments. London: Jessica Kingsley

Hopper, E and Weinberg, H (eds) (2011) The Social Unconscious in Persons, Groups and Societies, vol 1: Mainly Theory. London: Karnac Books

Nitsun, M (1996) The Anti-Group: Destructive Forces in the Group and their Creative Potential. London: Routledge

Nitsun, M (2015) Beyond the Anti-Group: Survival and Transformation. London: Routledge

Thompson, AE (1991) Freud's pessimism, the death instinct and the theme of disintegration in 'Analysis terminable and interminable'. International Review of Psycho-Analysis, 28, 165–180

Chapter 15

Traumatic Experiences

Restoring Mentalizing in Group Psychotherapies

Ulrich Schultz-Venrath

Introduction

Traumatic experiences and their treatments have a complex history. On the one side, traumatic experiences, which were detected in the families of the 19th century, were the origin and development of Freud's psychoanalysis. On the other side, psychoanalysis gained a certain reputation since its treatments of (social) traumata, especially of war neuroses, represented in the individual as "camptocormia" or functional bent back (Figure 15.1). More than 1 million soldiers should have been affected by these neuroses, including "shell-shock," "concussion neurosis" or "gas neurosis" in specialized hospitals during the World War I. The hospitals were established in Germany from 1916 to 1918 and frequently led by later known and famous psychoanalysts, e.g. Karl Abraham and Sandor Ferenczi. One of them was Ernst Simmel, who wasn't an analyst at that time but went through therapeutic experiences as a senior officer at a war neuroses hospital in Posen, in what is now Poland. After reading Freud's writings, Simmel developed special psychodynamic approaches that consisted regularly of an individual's "combination of analytic-cathartic pronunciation and dream interpretation," hypnosis and the use of other parameters, such as the use of "dummies" (for physically reacting to repressed emotions) (Simmel 1918, 1919). A "dummy" meant a puppet dressed up like an officer for the possibility of destroying it as a representation of the military superior. Looking back, it is amazing to see that throughout Simmel's clinical practice, he did NOT develop group therapy as one might think could easily come to mind. The term "active technique" was born, later to be criticized, which enabled Simmel to achieve exemption from the war neurotic symptoms in two or three sessions. These sessions proved to be more successful than electric and galvanic shock-treatments, which were frequently used by former psychiatrists. Simmel and Ferenczi did no longer understand traumatic neurosis as sequelae of sexual conflict, but as a severe regression to a phylogenetic and ontogenetic "proto-psyche" in which "states of excitement ... are simply dealt with by motor discharge" (Ferenczi 1919 [1984], p. 183). The primacy

DOI: 10.4324/9781003269649-21

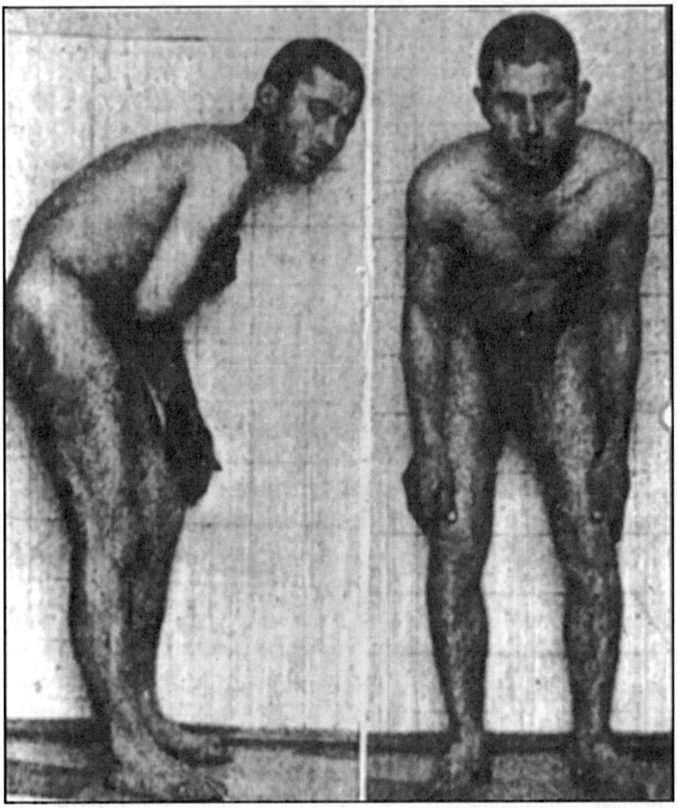

Figure 15.1 Camptocormia or functional bent back as a war neurosis in World War I (Souques & Rosanoff-Saloff 1915).

of sexuality in psychoanalysis shifted from the 1920s to the role of aggression, whereas Freud referred to a "natural aggression instinct," not existing primarily, but only as "descendant" of the death drive (Freud 1930a, p. 481).

This was also the context, in which the famous quotation of Freud was born: "It is very probable, too, that the large-scale application of our therapy will compel us to alloy the pure gold of analysis freely with the *copper of direct suggestion* [...] But no matter how psychotherapy is formed for the people, of which elements it may be composed, its most effective and important components will certainly remain those borrowed from strict, biasless psychoanalysis" (Freud 1919a, p. 194). With the disappearance of the symptoms of the war neuroses, the psychodynamic treatment was over. However, Ernst Simmel was aware that "an analytical cure of the entire personality, even with a condensed and combined methodology, [...] was reserved for the psycho-clinic of the future" (Simmel 1919, p. 43).

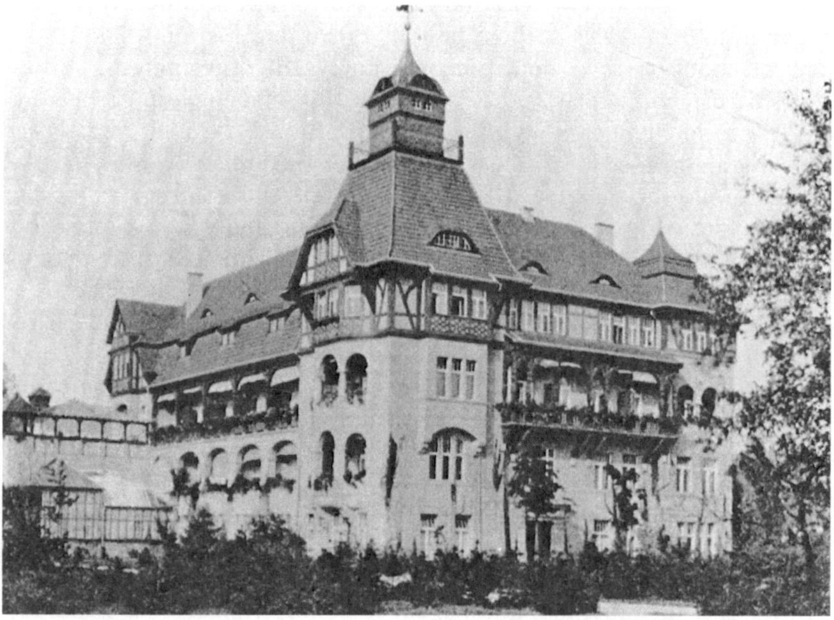

Figure 15.2 Psychoanalytic Clinic Sanatorium Schloss Tegel (1927–1931).

It's an interesting fact that Simmel together with Max Eitingon became then not only the founder of the first psychoanalytic polyclinic 1919 in Berlin, but also the founder of the first psychoanalytic hospital Sanatorium Schloss Tegel in 1927, a privately financed hospital with 70 beds in the north of Berlin (Figure 15.2).

Simmel knew that the clinic situation was not limited to the analyst-analysand relationship and offered his patients multiple transferences in the sense of an extended person of the analyst or the original family. Each morning, the nursing staff met with the doctors to discuss their observations outside the daily treatment hours on the couch and to receive rules of conduct for the following day from the analysts. Although he knew that at the same time, the housemother, physicians, nurses and fellow patients would have the role of a phantom for mother, brothers and sisters to reactivate the neurotic process, he didn't take the step toward group therapy or family therapy.

Surprisingly, however, there could well have been an encounter with a group concept in 1928: Ernst Simmel and Trigant Burrow—the latter used the term "group analysis" at first (without own experiences of war neuroses) published their treatment methods side by side in the German International Journal of Psychoanalysis, apparently without knowing each other (Burrow 1928b; Simmel 1928). Furthermore, the juxtaposition of both articles did not seem to have inspired other psychoanalysts. One reason could be that Freud and his followers weren't amused about Burrows' invention or discovery of group analysis—Ernest Jones described the newly elected American Psychoanalytic Association (APA) president Burrow in a letter dated May 27, 1925 as "very vague and muddle-headed" (Paskauskas 1993, p. 576); Simmel was, of course, a Freud-follower. The fact that Freud and his closest disciples did not become fans of Burrows' experiments of "group analysis" as a new tool in the treatment of neurotic or traumatized patients had an impact on Simmel's conception of the first psychoanalytic clinic, which had to be closed due to the global economic crisis in 1931. Nevertheless, it was the birth of a dual psychoanalytic inpatient treatment concept on the couch (Figure 15.3) for a range of mental disorders, including later so called post-traumatic disturbances, which then and now included a variety of mental and psychosomatic disorders to which trauma makes a remarkable transdiagnostic contribution.

Not only then, but still today, the ideas and theories concerning "trauma" or "traumatized person" are not sufficient to understand the complexity, which the refugee dilemma revealed (Varvin 2018; 2022). In the wake of individual and collective countertransference reactions, the word "trauma" is in danger of losing its theoretical grounding and

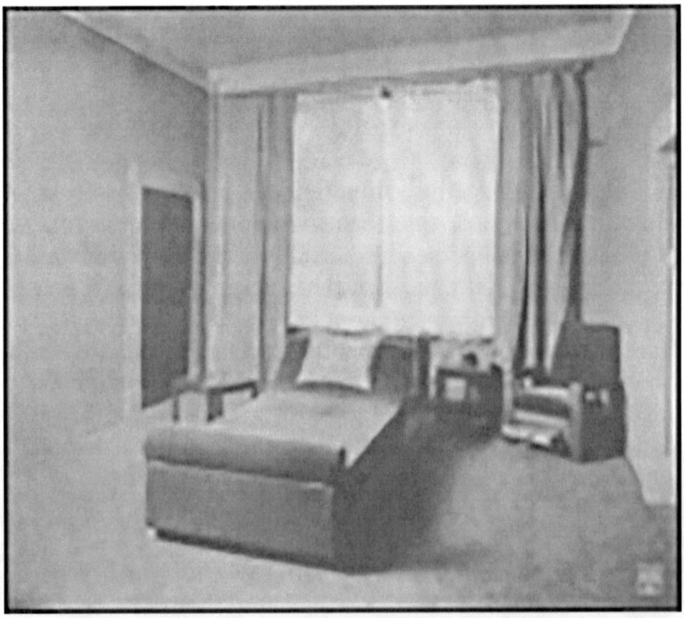

Figure 15.3 The treatment room in Sanatorium Schloss Tegel, 1927.

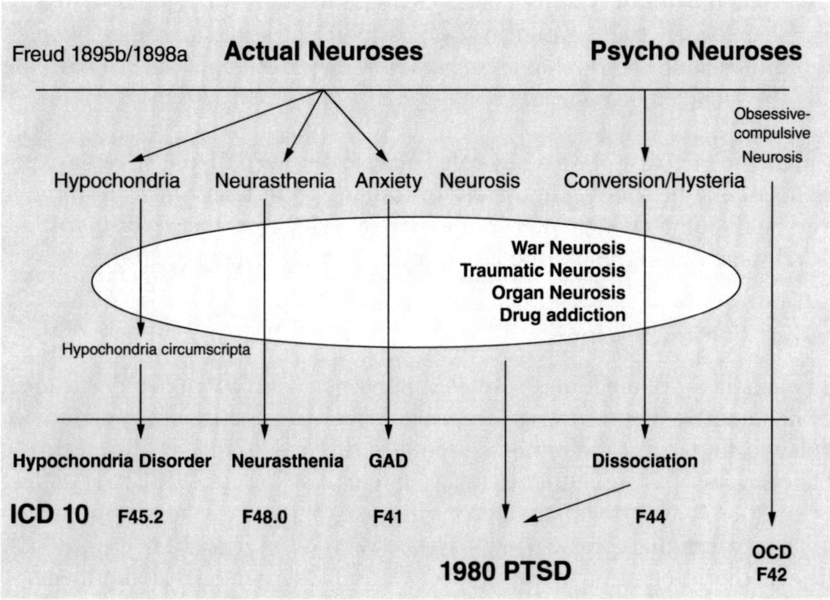

Figure 15.4 Historical taxonomy of diagnoses from Freud to ICD 10.

becoming the object of the projection of undefinable fears. If one speaks on "traumatic experiences" from a historical perspective, we should look on the history of taxonomy of diagnoses (Figure 15.4). Starting with Freud's epochal distinction between actual neuroses and psychoneuroses, the term posttraumatic stress disorder (PTSD) dates from a more recent period among many, sometimes overlapping with the wide range of medically unexplained symptoms and somatoform disorders. It is now legitimately argued by the founders of the mentalization model that trauma is best conceptualized as a transdiagnostic factor with a wide range of emotional and functional somatic illness problems. Against this background, the question remains "what is it that makes trauma potentially such a disruptive experience and so difficult to treat?" (Luyten & Fonagy 2019, p. 79).

Luyten and Fonagy (2019) try to answer this question, which refers also to the types of trauma (impersonal, interpersonal or attachment trauma) of Allen (2005) by three issues:

1 Traumatic experiences play a key role in the *regulation of distress and emotions*.
2 Such experiences result mostly in subsequent *problems in mentalizing*.

3 "The impact of trauma may contribute to *epistemic mistrust*—that is, the closing off the mind to the possibility of accessing other people's minds as safe and reliable sources of knowledge about how to navigate the social environment" (Fonagy et al., 2015).

Epistemic mistrust plays a key role because of internalizing adverse experiences, like factors "cannot rely on others," "undeserving" and "interpersonal guilt," which determines to some degree the severity of the development of psychopathology (Aafjes-Van Doorn et al., 2021).

What Is Mentalizing?

The magical or sometimes so-called nonsense word *mentalizing* is a form of imaginative mental activity, namely, perceiving and interpreting human behavior in terms of intentional mental states (e.g. needs, desires, feelings, beliefs, goals, purposes and reasons) (Bateman & Fonagy 2016). Every affect or emotion is intentional, that means disgust, for example, has the intentionality to externalize a toxic object. The power of this term as a new paradigm lies in the integration of self-reflective and interpersonal components—that's why it is very well suited as a construct in group contexts.

To develop the capacity of mentalizing is a long-lasting process over three to five years with integration of the implicit, semantic-episodic and autobiographic memory, from one-to-threeword-language and from simple to then complex narratives, which correlate with increasing capacity of mentalizing (Figure 15.5). Like waves for the pre-mentalistic modes, memories and representations are sometimes not so firmly structured as we think. Memories are neurobiologically represented in a functional network like the representations of self and object, of affects and emotions.

The triangular affect regulation has its empirical foundation in early attachment observations between the caregiver and the child. In a good caregiver-child relationship, the caregiver is confronted with the crying baby being in a state of agitation or catastrophic feelings. At its best, the caregiver should digest, resonate and express his emotions in a congruent, marked mirroring way to decrease the agitation. (NB: This is a little bit more than containment). If frequently marked and contingent mirroring of the baby (or patient) succeeds—in the first six months of life, mutual joy interactions can be observed up to 30,000 times (Emde 1992). If early development is embedded in a landscape of happiness, a representation of the dominating affect joy or of the joyful interaction as a whole will emerge. The baby is then able to use this representation to better deal with future upcoming emotional crises. Infants come to recognize their feelings by virtue of caregivers mirroring their emotional states in a complex fashion. This understanding is supported by late memory research, which doubts the specificity of post-traumatic memory in general (Greenshoot & Sun 2014).

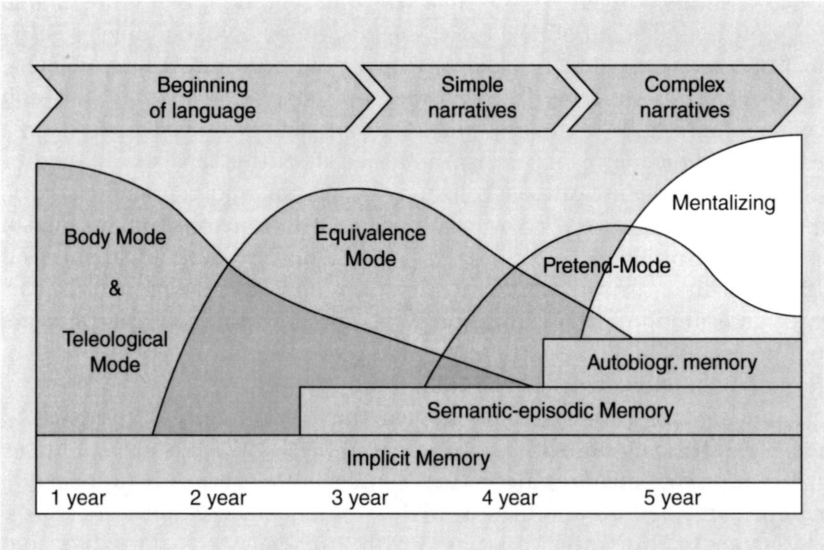

Figure 15.5 Memory, pre-mentalistic modes of affect regulation and development of language.

Repeating this experience of marked mirroring affects means to be concerned and helps the child, similar to the traumatized patient to advance from the body mode (Diez Grieser & Müller 2018; Schultz-Venrath 2021), which complements the previous three British working groups around Bateman and Fonagy. The body mode relates to the observation that pre- and postnatal, the baby cannot experience the body and psyche separately until around the ninth month. The baby is primarily concerned with his/her body and skin sensations. The traumatized adult patient similarly complains about physical symptoms as the only way to come into contact with an living object. The preverbal is dominant if any therapists can reach those patients only with "touching" words. All experiences are ultimately embodied, which in earlier times were known as part of the body-image or body-intercourse (see Paul Schilder, Judith Kestenberg, Maurice Merleau-Ponty). But even if it is meanwhile assumed that a certain "mentalizing" precedes language development, it is quite questionable whether the understanding of the child's inner state, which is experienced physically and communicated "pre-linguistically" long before the first word appears, should really already be called "embodied mentalizing" (Fonagy & Target 2007), because the body is not yet mentalized at this time. These phenomena can certainly be understood as an attempt to feel oneself in the absence of an object. Insofar, insecure or disorganized attachment experiences in early development as a result of early traumatization can lead to different attempts of self-assurance in case of unstable self-representation, like skin-picking, self-injuries, hyperembodiment in eating disorders, body building or chewing fingernails or nail beds, etc. If mirroring of affects doesn't succeed (e.g. the caregiver is suffering from postpartum depression or psychosis and can't resonate, fails to congest and isn't able to express her-/himself on a marked and/or contingent mirroring), then does this lead to an alien or false self or to the use of the whole body expressing undifferentiated affects and emotions (as we well know from patients with somatization and autism spectrum disorders)? It is an interesting fact that borderline patients and patients with antisocial personality disorders may have the problem of correctly interpreting facial expressions, but also problematic is that they are highly sensitive and quicker to respond to emotional facial expressions than normal without warning (Lynch et al., 2006).

Bateman and Fonagy (2004) started their empirically derived list of non-mentalistic modes with the teleological mode, which is defined by the observation that mental states as needs and emotions are only expressed in actions. Only actions and their available consequences count—not words. This mode is also "often associated with a tendency to externalize non-mentalized experiences (i.e., alien-self experiences), particularly in individuals with a marked history of trauma" (Luyten et al., 2019, p. 49). In contrast to the teleological mode, the body mode is more focused on the self, while the teleological mode is more focused on the object. The teleological mode in groups is sometimes connected with malignant mirroring, which has the potential to locate the detached part of one's own self onto the other.

From the perspective of the mentalization model it's an interesting question of whether the concept of the development of the self in early childhood (Figure 15.6) can be transferred into the treatment of trauma in a wider sense. The pivot of trauma symptomatology seems to be a crash of a congruent self, losing the differences of emotions and affects, sometimes flowing into a dissociation or depersonalization—the pretend mode in our mentalization model—with a lack of coherent autobiographic memory narrative.

How to Restore Mentalizing after Traumatic Experiences?

In the treatment of traumatization, however, group therapy still plays a subordinate role, even in the mentalization model. This may have to do with the fact that the history of group analysis or psychodynamic group psychotherapies itself has to do with traumatization. Freud was no friend of group therapy, as evidenced by his attitude toward Burrow, the first American psychoanalyst to discover the group as an important treatment tool. Despite recent efforts by Gatti Pertegato (1999; Gatti Pertegato & Pertegato 2013), Sandner (2003), Schultz-Venrath (2015) and others,

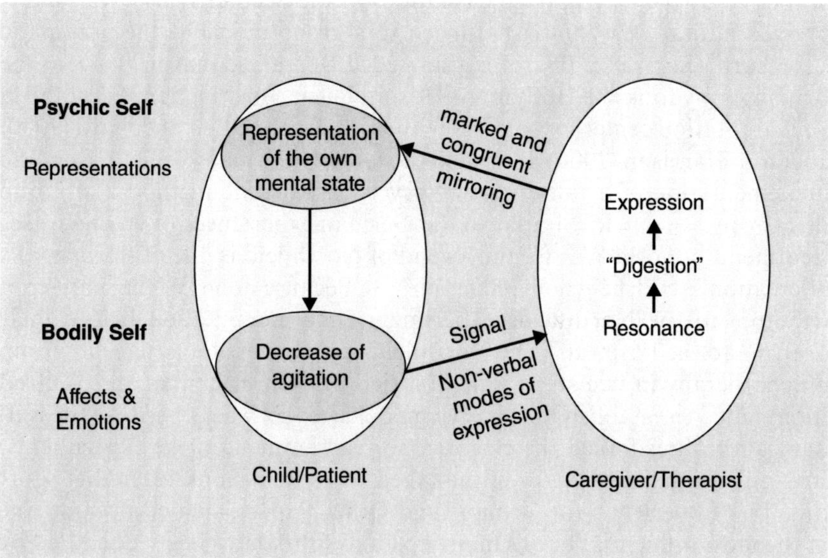

Figure 15.6 Affect regulation and the development of the Self (modified Fonagy et al., 2002 [2004]).

Burrow doesn't seem to be adequately valued today as a pioneer of group analysis in the group-analytic community. This is a gap in our recent history of group-analytic theory, possibly as a consequence of forced emigration of S. H. Foulkes, who had to reinvent himself in England. Burrow held the opinion "that no analysis of the individual could be complete without real study of the group of which he or she is a part. Further than this, he believed that mental disorders were problems of social relatedness and consequently that research could only be carried out in a group setting" (Burrow 1928a; Harrison 2000, p. 59). According to Burrow's perspective, conflicts showing a relational connotation, the quality of individual-environment interactions, is a determining factor in allowing or blocking the capacity to establish a subjective, constructive relationship with the world. In addition, he believed that in the course of subsequent life, groups could interfere with the individual's ability to cope with the imposition of serious life adversities. Such a concept was completely different from Freud's individualistic approach, which dealt with the instincts whose intrapsychic origins led to conflicts. Nevertheless, Burrow's work lacks the concept of treating (social) trauma in the group, possibly because he did not have to go to war.

Although the Adlerian Joshua Bierer "has a justifiable claim to be the pioneer of British group psychotherapy" (Harrison 2000, p. 54), World War II is viewed as the birth hour of group-analytic psychotherapy.

"Flooded by the traumatized casualities of the Second World War, hard-pressed military psychiatrists turned to a group model as the pragmatic [...] resort" (Barwick 2018, p. 3). It started at Northfield in April 1942, as the British Army took the Hollymoor Hospital near Birmingham to establish a rehabilitation center for soldiers with war neuroses. Ben Shephard (2000) and Tom Harrison (2000) described thoroughly the many difficulties of the implementation of a rather "new" psychotherapeutic method like group therapy in Northfield. Similar to the German experiences of war neuroses treatment in World War I, "the legend of Northfield is one of those myths of creation" (Hinshelwood 2000, pp. 7–8), because none "of the main contributors to the Northfields experiments had a reputation before their drafting to the hospital." The Northfield experiments took place in group psychotherapy in two steps. The first (led by John Rickman and Wilfred Bion) failed to establish a workable model after six weeks because the military authorities forced the closure and reassignment of the experiments. It is quite amazing that Bion managed to write a book after this short time on "Experiences in Groups: and Other Papers," which became one of the most influential books in group analysis to date. The second (led by Harold Bridger, Tom Main and S. H. Foulkes), learning in part from the previous cohort's mistake, fared better (Harrison 2000) even if Foulkes had to concede in his post-war memorandum "that group analysis, the most intensive form of group psychotherapy, isn't directly applicable in a military hospital" (Foulkes 2008; Schultz-Venrath 2008). He also had to concede that the mean short residence time of the war neurotic patients makes the processing of "deeper layers" impossible and calls for "modifications" of the technique, which are, according to Foulkes, less suitable for beginners. As we know from Tom Harrison, the patients received two individual sessions with Foulkes and one "closed" psychotherapy group per week: "In the latter work, Foulkes gave few instructions, sitting quietly most of the time. He talked to the group as a whole rather than to individuals and encouraged discussion about early childhood and dreams" (Harrison 2000, p. 195). This description of Foulkes' work differs a little bit from his theoretical work. It is also an interesting finding that the terms "trauma" or "post-traumatic disorder" do not appear in the book of Harrison's Northfield experiments any more than the term "regression" does. But even if the term "regression" would be of questionable benefit for the understanding of such group processes as Robi Friedman (2018) noted in his work on identity and soldiers matrix, the term "regression" doesn't exist in the texts of Foulkes and Harrison although clinical settings tend to promote dynamics of regression as Simmel (1928) had already described.

Like all trauma, "social" trauma also cannot be sufficiently understood and treated from only one perspective: "Clinical psychology and psychiatry describe individual and subjective pathology resulting from traumatic experience, and study the pathogenesis, coping mechanisms, and psychotherapeutic approaches" (Hamburger 2018, p. ix). In this sense, individual pathology is but one quite-limited perspective. On the other hand, social trauma—old wine in new bottles—is more than a diagnosis or disease—it is like a "concept," following Andreas Hamburger: "It is conceptualized from the start, when groups turn against groups, and when enacted, it is enacted as a specimen of a concept (like Auschwitz is a materialization of the concept of annihilation)." Independent of the many diagnostic trauma definitions, which are politically and chronologically determined, trauma is a subject where social and individual aspects are inseparably tied together. In group as in individual psychotherapies, traumatic experiences are also a discourse phenomenon. In the view of Jon Allen "trauma stems from repeatedly being left *psychologically alone in unbearable emotional pain*" (Allen 2013, p. xxii). Trauma is always an attachment trauma too. Exclusion from any group relationship is the worst case for every individual.

As I tried to contact the German Jewish emigres in the 1980s in the United States who were employees or members of the first psychoanalytic clinic in Berlin-Tegel, I was mostly confronted with epistemic mistrust, sometimes embedded in silence, then with an exchange in English before we landed in the Berlin dialect after a few or more days. These encounters are vividly stored in my memory. My countertransference reactions with cognitive and emotional symptoms are attenuated today in mentalization based group therapies by these experiences. These "traumatic shutdowns" (Laub 2017) described for individual therapies, but also happening in group therapies, often have a similar cycle: The voices of those affected begin to tremble, to stifle the language, if words can be found for the trauma at all, tears are flowing and not infrequently it has to be acted upon, e.g. by the patient leaving the group. First empirical results underlie the importance of focusing on increasing hope and perceived group affiliation in the treatment of personality dysfunction, because hopelessness at the beginning of treatment seems to moderate the effect of the outcome (Aafjes-Van Doorn et al., 2020).

The Role of the Conductor: To promote Mentalizing in Group Therapies with Traumatic Experiences

For traumatized patients it is difficult to develop trust in oneself and others when early relationships were not only insecure but also marked by traumatic attachment experiences. Assuming that impairing relationship experiences are usually also experienced in a group context and not only in a dyadic context - even the nuclear family of parents and siblings is a group - group psychotherapy offers a special opportunity to work on early shocks to the epistemic trust in the group. In this respect, there is a need for mentalization-based group psychotherapists to provide traumatized patients with special education regarding how to deal with the framework of the group and the group rules in order to minimize premature dropouts. This requires mentalization-based "dynamic administration". This is characterized by inviting the patient to come into affective exchange together about his (unconscious) fantasies, wishes, ideas and reservations about the groups. This is best achieved when the negative fantasies and mistrust in relation to the (unknown) group are explored particularly thoroughly and can be linked together with the underlying early, negative dyadic and group relationship experiences (Staun & Schultz-Venrath 2023).

The conductor of a group therapy has to work under pressure, exploring the patient's emotions and overall experience and verbalizing the patient's experience, preceding this with an ostensive cue. He has to develop a voice—an affective touching voice—starting with acknowledging "trauma:"

> I can see what you are getting at now (marked). You have made it so much clearer; that is really helpful (ostensive cue). Do you feel so hurt (emotion) that he does not notice how worried you are (context)? It seems to ignore it, leaving you thinking there is something wrong with you and you shouldn't be like that (effect).

On the other hand, the role of the therapist of a mentalization-based group (MBT-G) is not to ask the one who had just tried to talk about his or her trauma—his or her arousal is too high for mentalizing—but to ask the group if they know how the traumatized member feels or if they experienced something similar ("*How do you feel Mrs. X., what did Mr. B. tell us*?").

MBT-G-therapists are active, in collaboration with other group members, in the clarification of events. This active triangular turntaking is mostly a "no-go" for psychodynamic group therapists (Karterud 2015). MBT-G-therapists want to encourage detailed accounts of interpersonal events that are experienced by the individual members. They want the members' relational difficulties to be manifested in the here and now, spontaneously in the group processes. They allow, even encourage, themes to flow back and forth freely in an associative exchange of experiences, thoughts and feelings. This can be productive even if it comes at the expense of the possibility of detailed working through of crucial events like traumatic experiences. Mentalizing turntaking is an important part of the organizing principles of the group. The principle of turntaking in a wider sense guarantees to some degree that the patient who tells traumatic experiences cannot dominate and exploit the group in the reenactment of their trauma. Turntaking is an optimizing tool for the group as a training ground for mentalizing, not only at the beginning of a group. There is a good cause to conclude that early traumatization goes along with unstable representations in their procedural memory, formed either from an

Mode	Description
Body	Pre- and postnatal the baby can not experience body and psyche separately until around the ninth month. He/she is **primarily concerned with his/her body and skin** sensations.
Teleological	Mental states such as needs and emotions are expressed in action. **Only actions** and their available consequences **count** - not words.
Equivalent	**Outer world = inner world.** Mental states are experienced as real, as happens in dreams, flashbacks and paranoid delusions.
Pretend	Mental states are disconnected from reality. They retain a **sense of unreality** because they are not connected and anchored to reality.

Figure 15.7 Pre-mentalistic modes in the development of a child (Schultz-Venrath 2021).

exaggerated and overwhelmed (or vice versa: completely missing) mirroring of childish emotions caused by early caretakers. When representations are absent or fail to be linked together, this emerges as a type of prementalistic mode (Figure 15.7). Then, only dedicated therapeutic interactions accompanied by congruent mirroring processes can establish a mentalizing and ultimately reflective mode.

The body mode originally put forth by Diez Grieser and Müller (2018) and Schultz-Venrath (2021), presently an extension of the previous pre-mentalistic modes as earliest mode in the development of a baby, plays a particularly frequent role in group therapies in addition to the pretend mode, for example in the form of drinking, eating or special seating and so forth. This is followed by the teleological mode, which e.g. can occur in the form that the introduction of a new member "my name is Michael and I am being bullied" is answered by older group members with the words: "Shut the fuck up, Ingo!" A mentalising interaction by the group leader could be: "How do you think I would feel if you talked to me like that?" to draw aggression towards him or her.

The equivalent mode dominates the experience that the outer world correlates identically with the inner world. Mental states are experienced as real, similarly to dreams, flashbacks or paranoid delusions. The difference between imagination and reality is not developed or, if developed in this state, is broken down, whereas in the pretend "play" mode the inner world is decoupled from outer realities (Figure 15.7).

Patients in this mode trigger a sense of unreality because the inner world is not connected and anchored to reality, which is prevalent in histrionic and/or pseudo-mentalising patients..

Over time, a representation of the dominating affect or of interaction will emerge, which the baby or the traumatized patient in the group will use more and more to deal with emotional crises in the future and outside the group. Infants come to recognize their feelings by virtue of caregivers mirroring their emotional states in a complex fashion. This may also be due to insufficient mirroring in early childhood. For this assumption, Arcaro and coworkers (2017) reported that monkeys raised without exposure to faces did not develop face domains, although they showed normal retinotopic organization, indicating that early face deprivation leads to a highly selective cortical processing deficit.

Jacobson (1954) and later Winnicott have independently noted that internalizing the representation of the other before forming the boundaries of the self undermines the development of a coherent sense of self. The child is forced to internalize the other, not as an inner object but as a central part of his self (Fonagy 2008, p. 20), as a false or alien self. Such a false or alien self is extremely dependent of the behaviors and interpretations of the others, especially in the regulation of the six empirically derived primary affects related to the seeking-awarding-system, care (love), lust (sexual), fear, rage and – amazing for one or the other – play, even if a generally accepted definition of play doesn't exist (Figure 15.8).

Panksepp and Scott (2012) found that "one of the most commonly observed behaviors in young animals is their playfulness, specifically pouncing, chasing, wrestling and play biting." This activity, known as rough and tumble play, has received relatively detailed behavioral descriptions within the animal literature in comparison to human studies. Although the precise functions of physical play remain unspecified, it is likely essential for optimal childhood development, both body and mind, with many demonstrated benefits (Burgdorf et al., 2010, Brown & Vaughan 2010). Play allows "pretend" rehearsal for the challenges and ambiguities of life, a rehearsal in which life and death are not at stake. Panksepp and Scott (2012) proposed that play forms the backbone of young children's daily life through spontaneous social learning that enhances social interactions, promotes learning, and provides positive affect that may increase epistemic trust, attachment and psychological resilience. If group psychotherapy can be playful, with humor that engages rather than hurting or distancing, can solve problems by give-and-take between own and others' perspectives, describe their own experience rather than define other people's experience or intentions, convey "ownership" of their behavior rather than a sense that it "happens" to them, be curious about other people's perspectives and expect to have their own views extended by others, then

Li Gi (2nd century AD)	**Descartes (1649)**	**Ekman & Friesen (1972)**	**Mertens & Krause (1993)**	**Panksepp (1998) Panksepp & Biven (2012)**
			Interest	SEEKING
	Surprise	Surprise	Surprise	
Joy	Joy	Luck	Joy	**PLAY (JOY)**
Love	Love			CARE (LOVE)
Lust	Desire			LUST (SEXUAL)
Fear		Anxiety	Anxiety	FEAR
				PANIC (Separation Distress)
Hate	Hate	Anger	Rage	RAGE

Figure 15.8 Primary affects/emotions (Schultz-Venrath 2015 [2013]).

successful mentalizing has begun. Such patients are relaxed and flexible, not "stuck" in one point of view.

References

Aafjes-van Doorn, K., Kealy, D., Ehrenthal, J. C., Ogrodniczuk, J. S., Joyce, A. S. & Weber, R. (2020). The effect of hopelessness and perceived group compatibility on treatment outcome for patients with personality dysfunction. *The Journal of Nervous and Mental Disease*, *208* (9), pp. 677–682.

Aafjes-van Doorn, K., McCollum, J., Silberschatz, G. & Snyder, J. (2021). Assessing internalized beliefs: Development of the Pathogenic Belief Scale. *Development and Psychopathology*, *33* (1), pp. 96–108.

Allen, J. G. (2005). *Coping with Trauma: Hope Trough Understanding*. Washington DC: American Psychiatric Publishing.

Allen, J. G. (2013). *Restoring Mentalizing in Attachment Relationships – Treating Trauma with Plain Old Therapy*. Washington DC, London: American Psychiatric Publishing.

Arcaro, M. J., Schade, P. F., Vincent, J. L., Ponce, C. R. & Livingstone, M. S. (2017). Seeing faces is necessary for face-domain formation. *Nature Neuroscience*, *20* (10), pp. 1404–1412.

Barwick, N. (2018). The development of group analysis. The principle of interconnectedness. In Barwick, N. & Weegmann, M. (Eds.), *Group Therapy – A Group-Analytic Approach* (pp. 3–17). New York: Routledge.

Bateman, A. W. & Fonagy, P. (2004). *Psychotherapy for Borderline Personality Disorder. Mentalization Based Treatment*. Oxford, New York: Oxford University Press.

Bateman, A. & Fonagy, P. (2016). *Mentalization-Based Treatment for Personality Disorders – A Practical Guide*. Oxford: Oxford University Press.

Brown, S. & Vaughan, C. (2010). *Play—How it Shapes the Brain, Opens the Imagination, and Invigorates the Soul.* New York: Penguin Group.

Burgdorf, J., Kroes, R. A., Beinfeld, M. C., Panksepp, J. & Moskal, J. R. (2010). Uncovering the molecular basis of positive affect using rough-and-tumble play in rats: A role for insulin-like growth factor I. *Neuroscience*, *168* (3), pp. 769–777.

Burrow, T. (1928a). Biological foundations and mental methods. *British Journal of Medical Psychology*, *8*, pp. 49–63.

Burrow, T. (1928b). Die Laboratoriumsmethode in der Psychoanalyse, ihr Anfang und ihre Entwicklung. *Int Z Psychoanal*, *14*, pp. 375–386.

Diez Grieser, M. T. & Müller, R. (2018). *Mentalisieren mit Kindern und Jugendlichen*. Stuttgart: Klett-Cotta.

Emde, R. N. (1992). Positive Emotions for Psychoanalytic Theory: Surprises from Infancy Research and New Directions. In Shapiro, T. & Emde, R. N. (Eds.), *Affect: Psychoanalytic Perspectives* (pp. 5–44). Madison, CT: International Universities Press.

Ferenczi, S. (1919 [1984]). Hysterische Materialisationsvorgänge. Gedanken zur Auffassung der hysterischen Konversion und Symbolik. In Ferenczi, S. (Ed.), *Bausteine zur Psychoanalyse* (3rd ed., Vol. III, pp. 129–147). Bern, Stuttgart, Wien: Huber.

Fonagy, P. (2008). A genuinely developmental theory of sexual enjoyment and its implications for psychoanalytic technique. *Journal of American Psychoanalytic Association*, *56* (1), pp. 11–36.

Fonagy, P., Gergely, G., Jurist, E. L. & Target, M. (2002 [2004]). *Affect Regulation, Mentalization and the Development of the Self.* London; New York: Karnac.

Fonagy, P. & Target, M. (2007). Attachment and reflective function: their role in self-organization. *Development and Psychopathology*, *9*, pp. 679–700.

Fonagy, P., Luyten, P. & Allison, E. (2015). Epistemic petrification and the restoration of epistemic trust: A new conceptualization of borderline personality disorder and its psychosocial treatment. *Journal of Personality Disorders*, *29* (5), pp. 575–609.

Foulkes, S. H. (2008). Ein Memorandum zur Gruppenpsychotherapie von Major S.H. Foulkes, R.A.M.C., Specialist Psychiatrist Northfield Military Psychiatric Hospital – July 1945. *Gruppenpsychotherapie und Gruppendynamik*, *44*, pp. 222–235.

Freud, S. (1919a). Wege der psychoanalytischen Therapie. In *GW XII* (pp. 183–194). Frankfurt am Main: S. Fischer.

Freud, S. (1930a). Das Unbehagen in der Kultur. In *GW IVX* (pp. 419–506). Frankfurt am Main: S. Fischer.

Friedman, R. (2018). *Die Soldatenmatrix und andere psychoanalytische Zugänge zur Beziehung von Individuum und Gruppe*. Gießen: Psychosozial-Verlag.

Gatti Pertegato, E. (1999). Trigant burrow and unearthing the origin of group analysis. *Group Analysis*, *32*, pp. 269–284.

Gatti Pertegato, E. & Pertegato, G. O. (2013). *From Psychoanalysis to Group Analysis: The Pioneering Work of Trigant Burrow*. London: Karnac.

Greenshoot, A. F. & Sun, S. (2014). Trauma and Memory. In Bauer, P. J. & Fivush, R. (Eds.), *The Wiley Handbook on the Development of Children's Memory* (Vol. 2, pp. 774–803). New York: Wiley.

Hamburger, A. (Ed.). (2018). *Trauma, Trust and Memory – Social Trauma and Rconciliation in Psychoanalysis, Psychotherapy, and Cultural Memory*. London, New York: Routledge.

Harrison, T. (2000). *Bion, Rickman, Foulkes and the Northfield Experiments. Advancing on a Different Front*. London, Philadelphia: Jessica Kingsley.

Hinshelwood, R. (2000). Foreword. In Harrison, T. (Ed.), *Bion, Rickman, Foulkes and the Northfield Experiments – Advancing on a different front* (pp. 7–10). London, Philadelphia: Jessica Kingsley Publishers.

Jacobson, E. (1954). The self and the object world: Vicissitudes of their infantile cathexes and their influence on ideational affective development. *The Psychoanalytic Study of the Child*, *9*, pp. 75–127.

Karterud, S. (2015). *Mentalization-Based Group Therapy (MBT-G)*. Oxford: Oxford University Press

Laub, D. (2017). Traumatic Shutdown of Narrative and Symbolization: A Failed Empathy Derivative. Implications for Therapeutic Interventions. In Laub, D. & Hamburger, A. (Eds.), *Psychoanalysis and Holocaust Testimony. Unwanted Memories of Social Trauma* (pp. 43–65). London: Routledge.

Luyten, P. & Fonagy, P. (2019). Mentalizing and Trauma. In Bateman, A. & Fonagy, P. (Eds.), *Handbook of Mentalizing in Mental Health Practice* (2nd ed., pp. 79–99). Washington, D.C.: American Psychiatric Association Publishing.

Luyten, P., Malcorps, S., Fonagy, P. & Ensink, K. (2019). Assessment of Mentalizing. In Bateman, A. & Fonagy, P. (Eds.), *Handbook of Mentalizing in Mental Health Pracice* (pp. 37–62). Washington DC: American Psychiatric Association Publishing.

Lynch, T. R., Rosenthal, M. Z., Kosson, D. S., Cheavens, J. S., Lejuez, C. W. & Blair, R. J. R. (2006). Heightened sensitivity to facial expressions of emotion in borderline personality disorder. *Emotion*, *6* (4), pp. 647–655.

Panksepp, J. & Scott, E. L. (2012). Reflections on Rough and Tumble Play, Social Development, and Attention-Deficit Hyperactivity Disorders. In Meyer, A. L. & Gullotta, T. P. (Eds.), *Physical Activity Across the Lifespan, Issues in Children's and Families' Lives* (pp. 23–40). New York: Springer Science+Business Media.

Paskauskas, R. A. (Ed.). (1993). *The Complete Correspondence of Sigmund Freud and Ernest Jones 1908-1939*. London, England: The Belknap Press of Harvard University Press.

Sandner, D. (2003). Die Begründung der Gruppenanalyse durch Trigant Burrow - seine Bedeutung für die moderne Gruppenanalyse. In Pritz, A. & Vykoukal, E. (Eds.), *Gruppenpsychoanalyse. Theorie – Technik – Anwendung* (2, veränderte Auflage ed., pp. 135–160). Wien: facultas.

Schultz-Venrath, U. (2008). "Heute war ein historischer Augenblick der Psychiatrie, aber niemand weiß etwas davon" – Zu den Anfängen analytischer Gruppenpsychotherapie durch S. H. Foulkes im Northfield Military Psychiatric Hospital. *Gruppenpsychotherapie und Gruppendynamik*, *44*, pp. 215–221.

Schultz-Venrath, U. (2015 [2013]). *Lehrbuch Mentalisieren. Psychotherapien wirksam gestalten*. Stuttgart: Klett-Cotta.

Schultz-Venrath, U. (2015). Die Entdeckung der „Gruppenmethode in der Psychoanalyse" (1926) von Trigant Burrow – ein verhinderter Paradigmawechsel? *Gruppenpsychotherapie und Gruppendynamik*, *51*, pp. 7–17.

Schultz-Venrath, U. (2021). *Mentalisieren des Körpers*. Stuttgart: Klett-Cotta.

Shephard, B. (2000). *A War of Nerves. Soldiers and Psychiatrists 1914–1994*. London: Pimlico, Random House.

Simmel, E. (1918). Kriegsneurosen und "Psychisches Trauma". *Ihre gegenseitigen Beziehungen dargestellt auf Grund psycho-analytischer, hypnotischer Studien*. Leipzig München: Otto Nemnich.

Simmel, E. (1919). Zweites Koreferat: Die Psychoanalyse der Kriegsneurosen. In *Zur Psychoanalyse der Kriegsneurosen. Internationale Psychoanalytische Bibliothek Nr. 1* (pp. 42–60). Leipzig, Wien: Internationaler Psychoanalytischer Verlag.

Simmel, E. (1928). Die psychoanalytische Behandlung in der Klinik. *Internationale Zeitschrift für Psychoanalyse*, *14*, pp. 352–370.

Souques, M. M. & Rosanoff-Saloff, X. (1915). La camptocormie. Incurvation du tronc, consécutive aux traumatismes du dos et des lombes. Considérations morphologiques. *Revue Neurologique*, *27*, pp. 937–939.

Staun, L & Schultz-Venrath, U. (2023). Epistemisches Vertrauen, Misstrauen und Leichtgläubigkeit in Psychodynamischen Gruppentherapien. In Fonagy, P. & Nolte, T. (Eds.), *Epistemisches Vertrauen—Vom Konzept zur Anwendung in Psychotherapie und psychosozialer Beratung*. Stuttgart: Klett-Cotta.

Varvin, S. (2018). Unser Verhältnis zu Flüchtlingen: Zwischen Mitleid und Entmenschlichung. *Psyche – Zeitschrift für Psychoanalyse und ihre Anwendungen*, *72* (3).

Varvin, S. (2022). *Psychoanalysis in Social and Cultural Settings. Upheavals and Resilience*. London, New York: Routledge.

Part VI

Pandemics and the Outer World Traumatic Impact

Chapter 16

The Child, the Adolescent and the Therapist

Playing and the Pandemic Reality

Eftychia-Evie Athanassiadou

When I try to describe my professional experience as a psychotherapist working in the pandemic, it seems impossible to differentiate it from my personal experience, as for the first time, my attitude and therapeutic decisions were massively affected by my own feelings about a traumatic external reality. For my generation, it was the first time that we had to face a worldwide life-threatening situation that no one knew exactly what to do or how and when we would get through it. My own immediate thought was that, like my ancestors survived war, I would also find a way to survive. My true reaction, however, was one of shock and terror in the images of massive deaths in Europe, hospitalizations, and the uncertainty of not knowing. So, at first, I had to find a way to survive, to bear the unthinkable, before I could "take the responsibility" to work through this traumatic situation with my patients. If this kind of threat was so disruptive for adults, how was it experienced by children and adolescents? Thinking back, I believe that MY most important concern was knowing that I could not be the therapist I was before, that is, a stable containing mother or firm father and, most importantly, I could not be neutral (as much as I could be before). I was there in the storm with them, not knowing much and, often, frightened as a child. So, we were now at the same place, therapists, children and parents. Above all this, I could not even offer the security and stability of our setting, my office, their play material, my live presence (in the first lockdown). Later, when we could meet again, I would realize that even this meeting in person was quite different from before since the masks and the social distancing measures had changed the therapeutic relationship and the way we could work. But most of all, it has changed our sense of omnipotence. Despite all my hesitations, I thought that even though this would definitely be a compromised, "different" psychotherapy, I made the choice to stay connected with my patients, taking into account of course the individual capacities and needs.

My previous experience as director of a phone helpline for children and adolescents proved to be valuable when the pandemic came into our lives. Two simple facts from my former experience encouraged me to decide to

DOI: 10.4324/9781003269649-23

continue working online. First, the accessibility of the online medium and the familiarity for children and adolescents (much more than me). Second, my own previous experience with adolescents online. However, I never before performed online psychotherapy for children and I must admit that at the beginning, thinking about the setting, the use of play, the need for the presence of the therapist especially for some pathologies, seemed an impossible task.

Considering children who had been in psychotherapy with me, I tried to follow a few basic principles. As I communicated with other colleagues either in the European Federation for Psychoanalytic Psychotherapy (EFPP) group or the Hellenic Society of Child and Adolescent Psychoanalytic Psychotherapy (HACAPP, Greek) to find support on how to procced, I decided to make a new "contract" with the child and family, as to assess their will and ability to cooperate and of course to explain the new "setting." Three main principles were, in my mind, important to keep in online psychotherapy:

1 The safeguarding of a "safe" confidential space for the child or in case the child was unable on his own, to assess the will and ability of the child to be in the "supervision" of parents.
2 The need to keep some aspects of the previous setting constant (the play materials in the room, my office room). In the process, I realized that it was important that the child also have a box in their own place that would resemble the therapy box and they could keep all of the play material of the sessions, with the prospect to merge the contents when we could meet again.
3 Assessment if that new medium would be fit for the needs of every single child or family separately.

So, I remember driving to my office with these terrible images in my mind, not seeing anyone on the street. As I thought, my office, the boxes with the toys and the internal setting as one would say, was from then on, my new frame along with my computer. What surprised me most was the fact that most of the children and adolescents were very eager to meet with me on the screen and were very active in the process, as this was for the first time in their own control. It seemed that for most of them it was a familiar "place" to be without their parents. A boy that I will soon describe in more detail even expressed the feeling that he was more comfortable online, as he finally could "come" on his own instead of his parents "telling" him to come.

However, this motivation and therapeutic alliance that was so strong at first, maybe as a reassurance that we are both alive and we have not been "destroyed" by the virus or in a more unconscious level by their aggressive or erotic fantasies, seemed for some children and adolescents to fade gradually. Especially for younger children or others with more primitive ego functioning, the absence of the physical body, of the reassurance of the presence of the other, the absence of touch, eye contact and smell, seemed in time to affect the trust and security of the therapeutic relationship.

More specifically, I will focus on four aspects of the therapeutic work:

1 Acknowledging the absence of the body presence of the therapist and its effects.
2 The specificities of transference and countertransference.
3 Playing as a way of making sense of the unthinkable.
4 Adolescents and the pandemic: A developmental conflict.

Acknowledging the Absence of the Body Presence of the Therapist and Its Effects

It is well supported that the presence of the body in psychotherapy is of the outmost importance as much of the unconscious communication can be through the soma (Lemma 2017). The bodily experience of the therapist and patient is therefore a reference to the primary relationship and an important source of information through transference and countertransference for the therapist. This view is even more pivotal when we are talking to children or adolescents, where the relationship with the parents and all the childhood conflicts and traumas are present in the here and now. So, we have to ask ourselves what kind of presence we were offering. Did we underestimate *the "loss"* of the embodied therapist and the live psychotherapeutic relationship? It is my hypothesis that for this virtual presence of the therapist to be "good enough," a child or adolescent should have been able to internalize the relationship with the therapist, which implies a good symbolic function and a preceding therapeutic relationship of sometime before moving to the screen. Younger children (4–6 years old) were the ones, in my experience, with the fewer resistances in speaking out their sense of loss and grief for what had been lost in the therapeutic relationship.

The therapist, too, as many before have described, (Russell 2019), finds him/herself trying to compensate for this loss of perceptual signals by trying hard to keep concentration and often in effect, losing the ability for having a "free floating attention" and "reverie." Further, many therapists, as myself, found themselves unable to stay silent due to the anxiety that through the screen it is difficult to "reach" the other.

Clinical examples

A 7-year-old girl joins the online session and plays with her dolls. As I comment on play she asks me: Can you see my dolls? Can you feel their hair? She also constantly "plays" with the idea that even though I can see her I cannot really "feel" her through my senses. She finally tells me: "If you cannot feel the water that I will spill on you then you are not really present."

What she seems to imply is that in order for her to acknowledge my presence, she needs to trust that we experience the same things at a sensory level.

Luc, aged 4, looks at me through the screen surprised and a little angry. He listens carefully when I am telling him that I am in the office where we meet. I show him the toys and his box. He first talks about a good dream with a dog eating a bone while he plays with his grandmother. Then a bad dream. A crocodile that threatens to bite him and then falls off the cliff. I remind him of the crocodile of our meetings and he asks me to pull out the rope and tie him as we often do in order to save him from falling. I take off the rope and tie it. He then begins to build a road. This road has many obstacles, but bridges are built that allow people to pass through rivers and shattered roads. The road seems to be without end. I notice that, as I tell him that it also reminds me what we have been going through these few months. Due to this virus no road can take us where we want. It has no end. He finally arrives at the mall. But then he cannot go inside because of the coronavirus. I ask him what he thinks of the virus. He goes under the table for a few minutes. He seems scared. He finally comes back saying that the virus is bad for our body because it is dirty.

Luc through his dreams and his symbolic play talks in parallel for the internal as well as the external reality. It is evident that the virus has triggered primitive oral anxieties along with the fear of intrusion and annihilation. The "good dream" represents the old days where Luc could meet with his grandmother and her dog. This image is followed by the "bad dream" where all this blissful caring is gone due to a dangerous crocodile (virus) that threatens him with intrusion and death. In the end, however, the crocodile falls, but this solution does not reassure him. In this moment there is an intersection with the internal reality of Luc as his own aggressiveness is projected on the crocodile who in play we have to contain and "save." In this way, he is able to "connect" with split-off parts of himself and feel integrated. When this internal "connection" is possible, the roads and bridges of play are expressing the processing of all these different aspects of the fears about the virus, the mourning about the loss, and the longing for "connecting" once more and relating with the object- therapist. As we can "make sense" through the symbols, Luc can go on to present another fear associated with the external but also the internal reality of an Oedipal boy. The fear of exclusion, the closed doors of the parental couple and the feeling that his longing to go in and his anger for not being able to, is something dirty even dangerous. In the pre-COVID time, we often discussed his fantasies, as in play he fought and killed the male animal to have the female for himself.

Second lockdown

September of 2020, we are back again for a while. Children go back to school, but soon after, there is a lockdown again. I meet Luc on the screen once more.

He cries inconsolably because he won't go on climbing lessons for a while. Father says, "Why can't you accept it?" He builds a boat but soon turns back to wanting to see the teacher. I feel he is mourning. Dad says we're going to build a climbing wall in the house but that doesn't comfort him either. He says: "I want the same teacher, the same wall, ***alive****." This last word shatters me. I suddenly feel like I want to cry with him. Is he afraid that we could probably all die, or is he talking about his feeling that what we offer him as an alternative (therapy, play) is not "alive" for him? My own losses and the grieving that I did not do, go through my mind. He expresses it. Dad is desperately trying to provide solutions manically. Finally, I say to both of them: "It' s all right to cry since It's very hard to miss out on so many important things and people you love. Even* ***we*** *can't meet in person."*

He suddenly stops crying and listens carefully. He starts building a boat which will take people to the different islands if it survives the dangerous fish in the water. After the session I feel wound out. I wonder: who will be able to contain the mourning for the losses of this child? The mourning of all of us? Are we able to mourn right now or is it too early? On the other side, can the bridges and boats be a symbol of the bridges we are trying to build through the screen in order to keep the "connection" alive?

Countertransference Issues in Child Psychotherapy During the Pandemic

Kohon (2020), in a recent article about countertransference wonders:

> How might the uncertain reality of the pandemic affect this use of the countertransference, particularly in relation to a changed setting and a potentially compromised paternal function that complicates attempts to differentiate our own anxieties and defenses from the patient's?

The above example of Luc, I think, is one that pictures clearly one of the transference and countertransference problems present in our work during the pandemic. On the one hand, there is the complex interplay between the fantasies, especially those related with aggressiveness and primitive annihilation anxieties, and an external reality where the terror of harming people, fear of intrusion and need to stay away from human contact are making these fantasies possible. We as therapists also stay away from our child and adolescent patients in order to protect them and ourselves. But what does this "mean" for them? Are we afraid of them? Of their aggressive or sexual intrusions?

I believe that this complication in countertransference, even though acknowledged before the pandemic, in this instance more than ever, presented for me much more than before a need for the therapist to have a "third" in the equation. That means a space where all this dread and trauma of myself and the patients can be expressed, contained and find its personal meaning. For me, this function was performed by supervision and group discussion with colleagues.

Going on to the issue of **adolescent psychotherapy** in the pandemic, I will address two main issues. One has to do with the obvious: adolescent developmental needs are in complete opposition with the reality of the pandemic. Socialization, autonomy from the family, sexuality and proximity were all restricted and even more, described as "dangerous" for the self and the other. Winnicott (2017) refers to the adolescent who in order to become an adult has to go through the death and the "murder" of the parents. In the pandemic this "murderous" fantasy could become actual. Many adolescents went out to meet their friends without masks knowing that their older-aged or sick parents could be at risk.

An adolescent girl in the second lockdown goes out secretly to meet her friends in their house. Going back, her parents ask her where she has been and if she wore her mask. Her father is an overweight man who is much afraid of the virus. The family drama emerges.

As the mother tries to take the part of the daughter the father explodes: "Are you trying to kill me? Do you understand that my life is in danger because of you? Are your friends more important than my life?"

As guilt was one of the most relevant feelings along with fear of dying, I found that many adolescents could not psychically survive this conflict. The result was either a depressive position where guilt and the fear of harming the others along with annihilation fears prevailed, or a defensive position of dissociation, refusal and acting out. As a therapist, I often found myself quite worried about adolescent patients.

On the opposite side, although adolescents were so prone to act on this impulsiveness so typical of this phase, others were able to use the mediated therapy to be contained and find meaning.

A late adolescent boy starts online sessions in the pandemic. In the previous in person psychotherapy, the boy is very shy and feels awkward with his body. He has no eye contact and is mostly silent. He never refers to romantic relationships. The therapist hypothesizes that there could be some erotic transference to the therapist.

The distance of the screen on the online meetings seems to facilitate the adolescent into expressing his fantasies and erotic impulses in a "safe space" without the threat of acting out. This "third space" has been conceptualized as the "e-third" (Stadter 2012). Scharff (2012) refers to the safety of distance that allows certain affective states that may previously have been withheld or dissociated to emerge. She associates this with the fact that distance protects from impulsive action.

However, as Stadter notes, the e-third is interfering in the relationship between two people, especially with intimacy and reflection, in contrast with the analytic third of Ogden (2018), where the intersubjective space promotes reflection and intimacy. I think that in the presented situation, the notion of the third in COVID as well as on the screen is an important one. COVID reality disproved the symbiotic fantasy. We are no longer "safe" in the presence of the other. For us therapists, the screen became the barrier between us and our patients. In this distance however, some were able to find the "optimal distance" (Akhtar 2019), whereas others cultivated the illusion of symbiotic even pervert fantasies.

In conclusion, I couldn't resist sharing a very moving moment from the therapy of a 11-year-old girl that, through play, I think represents all that has been lost and found in these peculiar times, like distance and togetherness and the need of children for "being with the other" in order to survive psychically and develop. I must admit that children and adolescents, through their liveness, playfulness and hope, even from a distance, helped me understand and experience the essence of the therapeutic relationship in a time of threat, as this relationship was strengthened by our effort to overcome this distance.

Mary takes a surgical glove and makes a baby by blowing air in it and drawing eyes and mouth. She comes and puts it in my arms in order to take care of it. I say that she would like me to hold her like the baby glove, but she is afraid to come close to me. She takes back the baby and tries to cut it with the scissors. It has been injured but it will live. She puts tape on the holes. In the end, she puts it in her box and asks me to watch over. The next session is online one due to her being in contact with the virus. She admits that she is afraid and cannot sleep at night, thinking that some part of her body will fall off. She then asks me if I took care of her baby glove and asks me to show it to her through the screen. She puts her head so close, like she wants to pass through the screen and reach me. When she is reassured that the baby is ok in my arms, she tells me the following story:

> *I want to tell you about a movie. It's called "Stranger Things."*
>
> *It's a scary movie but I can survive it. A child disappears and enters the world of upside down. It is a world where only shadows remain; it is a world where you are neither dead nor alive. What a strange world!*

References

Akhtar, Salman. *Turning Points in Dynamic Psychotherapy: Initial Assessment, Boundaries, Money, Disruptions and … Suicidal Crises*. Routledge, London, 2019.

Christogiorgos, Stylianos, and Georgios Giannakopoulos. "Online Psychodynamic Psychotherapy for Children and Adolescents: Challenges and Questions." *Child and Adolescent Psychodynamic Psychotherapy*, Nova Science Publishers, New York, 2021.

Kohon, Sebastian. "Challenges to Making Use of Countertransference Responses during the Covid-19 Pandemic – Some Preliminary Thoughts." *Journal of Child Psychotherapy*, vol. 46, no. 3, 2020, pp. 283–288, https://doi.org/10.1080/0075417x.2021.1898043.

Lemma, Alessandra, and Luigi, Caparrotta. *Psychoanalysis in the Technoculture Era*. Routledge, London, 2014.
Lemma, Alessandra. *The Digital Age on the Couch: Psychoanalytic Practice and New Media*. Routledge, London, 2017.
Ogden, Thomas H. "The Analytic Third: Working with Intersubjective Clinical Facts." *The Analytic Field*, 2018, pp. 159–188, https://doi.org/10.4324/9780429481031-9.
Russell, Gillian Isaacs. Screen Relations: *The Limits of Computer-Mediated Psychoanalysis and Psychotherapy*. Routledge, London, 2019.
Scharff, Jill Savege. "Clinical Issues in Analyses over the Telephone and the Internet." *The International Journal of Psychoanalysis*, vol. 93, no. 1, pp. 81–95, 2012, https://doi.org/10.1111/j.1745-8315.2011.00548.x.
Stadter, Michael. *Presence and the Present Relationship and Time in Contemporary Psychodynamic Therapy*. Jason Aronson, Lanham, MD, 2012.
Widdershoven, Marie-Ange. "Clinical Interventions via Skype with Parents and Their Young Children." *Infant Observation*, vol. 20, no. 1, pp. 72–88, 2017, https://doi.org/10.1080/13698036.2017.1378528.
Winnicott, D. W. *Playing and Reality*. Routledge, London, 2017.
Wu, Tianchen, et al. "Prevalence of Mental Health Problems during the COVID-19 Pandemic: A Systematic Review and Meta-Analysis." *Journal of Affective Disorders*, vol. 281, pp. 91–98, 2021, https://doi.org/10.1016/j.jad.2020.11.117.

Chapter 17

Estrangement and Intimacy in the Time of Zoom

Mary Morgan

In "Civilization and its Discontents," Freud declared that "At the height of being in love the boundary between ego and object threatens to melt away. Against all the evidence of his senses, a man who is in love declares that 'I' and 'you' are one, and is prepared to behave as if it were a fact" (1930, p. 66). If this 'being in love' state continued endlessly for couples, then perhaps lockdown in the context of a pandemic would have been a welcome phenomenon. And indeed, some couples have found closeness during lockdown, anywhere on a continuum from a retreat to merger, to a healthier development of their intimacy or a re-finding of lost intimacy. But for other couples, lockdown has created a lack of psychic space that has not been easy to manage. The conscious and unconscious arrangements couples make to manage the nearness and distance in their relationship, has been disrupted and recalibrated in ways beyond their control. Lack of physical space, the whole family at home and a hostile external outside world has only exacerbated these difficulties.

George Elliot, in her classic novel, "Middlemarch" said, "Marriage is so unlike anything else. There is something even awful in the nearness it brings" (quoted by Cohen in the Guardian, 2021, p. 22). The 'nearness' of the other, experienced in the recent pandemic, can be extremely challenging. The blind spots the couple have about the other, their capacity to 'turn a blind eye,' has been tested as the other comes into closer focus. While, for some, this has led to development in their relationship, for others it has had a destabilising effect as there is no escape from those unwanted and avoided aspects of the other.

Cohen suggests the essential paradox of intimacy is:

> That in intensifying our closeness to another, we not only make them more familiar to us; we come alive to their strangeness and irreducible difference.
>
> (2021, p. 23)

DOI: 10.4324/9781003269649-24

In the normal life cycle of a couple, the process of disillusionment is lived out in everyday life. The other and the couple's relationship are gradually brought into more contact with reality. The idealised version of the other and of the relationship is revealed to be different—not all that it was imagined to be, or what was thought to be needed. The other can meet some of our needs but is unable, or chooses not to, meet others. Their 'nearness' brings the discovery that they are, in fact, a challenging mixture of things. Again, one can see that the nearness brought on by lockdown is potentially a growth point for a couple, seeing and coming to terms with aspects of the other previously avoided through the arrangements the couple have made to live their lives. But for others, it has become closer to a claustrophobic nightmare, as the other is felt to intrude upon the psychic space of the self.

Colman (2014) in his paper, "The Intolerable Other: the Difficulties in Becoming a Couple" argues that along with our basic need to seek an object, being in a relationship brings an anti-relating part of us—an inherent antipathy toward the other and their difference from ourselves. This idea has been expressed by other writers, notably the late Janine Puget, who stated:

> To work with the complexity of links as it happens with family and couple psychoanalysis has to do with the difficulty to accept the unavoidable otherness and alienness of each one."
>
> (2019, p. 25)

As well as the difficulty in facing 'difference' in the close confinement of lockdown, there is an issue of psychic space. Colman suggests that as well as need to relate, we also have a basic need for 'non-relating.' He stresses this is different from 'anti-relating,' a narcissistic turning away from the other. He says, "non-relating refers simply to the need for 'space' and solitude and is an inherent—and essential—aspect of all relationship. Relating to others is only tolerable within certain limits—beyond these we speak of 'intrusion' and 'invasion,' an abrogation of our autonomy."

The problem is that what is necessary space to one partner may be experienced as rejection, loneliness, and isolation to the other one. There may be differences between the partners in their 'capacity to be alone' (Winnicott, 1958), one of them feeling alone in the presence of a secure internal object while for the other, being alone feels like abandonment. At the same time, 'closeness' to one of the partners might feel like a claustrophobic takeover to the other. These differences in the need, or capacity for non-relating, and as Winnicott (1958) described, "the capacity to be alone," can lead to very difficult 'anti-relating' dynamics in the couple. One partner's expression of their needs and differences can feel to the other as an intrusive act from which they have to turn away or retaliate. The couple can feel there is not enough space in the relationship for them both, nor is there any space outside the relationship, such as the usual ventures to work, exchanges with work colleagues, or dropping the children at school and encountering other parents. The couple are together all the time, and with the children at home being home schooled, a claustrophobic atmosphere can develop that feels unbearable. During the pandemic lockdowns, there have been many reports of escalating disturbing dynamics in couple relationships which are difficult for the couple and the analyst to contain. The analyst's capacity for containment has been affected by the disruptions to the setting and the limitations of working remotely.

The claustrophobic lack of space in the couple's relationship also has an impact on the couple's capacity to process their feelings and to think. The couple's capacity to take a 'third position' (Britton, 1989) on their relating is an important internal resource in a relationship, especially at times of stress (Morgan, 2001, 2019). I have described this capacity as a 'couple state of mind,' a capacity provided by the couple analyst which, over time, can be internalised into the couple relationship. During times of immense stress, such as that experienced in a global pandemic, this capacity in a relationship is all the more important. However, if the pandemic has boldly reminded us of anything, it is the interrelationship between the internal and the external. A couple state of mind is about finding an internal position, a third perspective, on what is occurring in the relationship between oneself and the other. But this process of being able to psychically move to a different place in one's mind might be supported by being able to move physically away from the other into a different and less claustrophobic space. This might be through engaging with colleagues and work mates, friends, family and the other perspectives that the outside world offers. Without this, it is still possible to find a couple state of mind, but it might be a lot more difficult, especially for those couples for whom this capacity is not securely in place.

Estrangement and Intimacy in the Therapeutic Situation

While couples have been struggling with unexpected challenges to their relationships, they have also had to manage without the usual form of containment in their therapy. It has been interesting to me how the nearness and distance in the online setting has impacted the work. At the beginning, I think most of us expected that what we would be dealing with was the disruption to the setting and particularly the distance and the loss of not being physically present with our patients.

In this online analytic world, the physical aspect of the frame has had to be provided by the patients themselves, even though part of our job has been to help them think about how to establish this. Finding a suitable setting to meet for the online sessions has been difficult for some who have been unable to find a private space in their home. Some have had to go and sit in their car—with one patient having to drive off several times in the session persecuted by traffic wardens. Others, particularly young people in shared housing, have had to move outside and find a quiet park bench and then there is a question about how confidential a space can be created and if the therapist can agree to it. Times like this are hard for the patient and hard for the therapist to feel as if there *is* a setting in which the work can take place.

Our patients are also deprived of the experience of the consulting room, waiting room, bathroom, and the tactile and sensory experiences of entering the analyst's physical space, symbolic of her containing mind. There is no journey to the session in which associations and thoughts might arise nor a post-session journey in which the session is processed in some way or another. It is hard to imagine that this does not affect the patient's experience of being taken in by the analyst and that the space to process the analytic work isn't compromised. This is another example of the how important the movement from being inside an analytic space to being outside it can be in the process of reflection and psychic growth.

Having tried like others to replicate the in-person setting as much as possible online, I started to accept that it was a compromised setting and drew on other such experiences of this in the past.

It helped me to remind myself that not all analytic work takes place in the analyst's consulting room. I remembered a conversation I had many years ago with Moses Laufer, who was one of the psychoanalysts who set up the Brent Consultation Centre in London, now a world-renowned clinic providing analytic therapy for young people. He told me that at the beginning, some adolescents could not sit in the consulting room for 50 minutes. He decided to meet with them in their surroundings, for example around a snooker table, playing snooker with them. That was where the analytic work began. It also brings to mind a Family Centre I worked in as a social worker, in which I consider much analytic work took place. But arriving to work with a couple or a family, one sometimes found the room hadn't been booked, or someone else was in it. It took time to arrange the chairs and establish the boundary but even then, it wasn't perfect, in fact even without a pandemic, the setting never is, as John Churcher points out:

> In practice, we all have to cope every day with the fact that the setting we maintain is not ideal. It is constantly being compromised, infringed upon, and modified. Patients may attack it; colleagues undermine it; we ourselves neglect it. Like the house you live in, it only survives because you also care for it and try to repair the damage as you go along.
>
> (Churcher, 2005, p. 9)

These experiences and ideas helped me accept that this was the new compromised setting and that was what had to be worked with both in the bigger picture, for example, the ongoing loss of the consulting room, real and symbolic, the anxiety about the therapist's health and survival and so on, and in the minutiae—how some patients wanted me to send a Zoom invite for each session, even though my Zoom contact stayed the same, because as I understood it, it symbolised me opening the door and inviting them in to the consulting room.

Perhaps the most fundamental way that the external setting is comprised is that the analyst can't take care of it in the usual way that Churcher describes. The patient having to manage the setting themselves affects how they can be in the session. One could say they need more ego strength to hold together what the analyst would normally be responsible for holding. This may have unconsciously impacted what they can bring to their session.

The change in setting has also had a profound impact on the analyst, especially for those who have had to change their physical setting. It reminds us just how important the external setting is in supporting our internal analytic setting. The internal setting can be defined as "the capacity to hold oneself at a level of listening specifically directed towards understanding the patient's unconscious" (Civitarese, 2005, p. 1300). It has been argued that that if the analyst's internal setting is secure, then it is possible to manage flexibility in the external setting. Parsons has elaborated this idea:

> Just as the external setting defines and protects a spatiotemporal arena in which patient and analyst can conduct the work of analysis, so the internal setting defines and protects an area of the analyst's mind where whatever happens, including what happens to the external setting, can be considered from a psychoanalytic viewpoint. The external setting may be breached from the outside if, for example, the builders next door start hammering or someone accidentally enters the room; or from the inside if the patient acts out in certain ways or the analyst does something to disrupt it. But if the analyst's internal setting remains intact, infringements of the external setting can still be thought about in terms of their analytic significance and brought within the analysis.
>
> (Parsons, 2007, p. 1444)

Analysts have described how they have, and have not, been able to maintain an internal setting. Some, perhaps many, as Parsons describes, have found a way of maintaining their internal setting and working analytically with the disruptions to the external setting, as material, in the way I have described above. However, many have found this much more challenging, at least some of the time, and have been feeling something important is missing. They feel they are not able to provide what their patients need and are not doing a very good job. Some patients have found the changed external setting more difficult than others and for some analysts the internal setting has felt quite shaky. Given the emotional impact of the pandemic on our patients and ourselves, and the major disruption to the external setting at a time that its consistency and reliability is most needed, it is likely that our internal setting has been harder to maintain. After all, some analysts in order to be able to work remotely have had the de-stabilising experience of having to relocate and establish a new external setting. As Bridge points out, the relationship between the external setting and the internal setting can be considered a reciprocal one. She says, "the external frame functions as a support to the internal setting and that, if it stretched too far, the internal setting can be damaged" (2013, p. 484). Perhaps for most of us there has been a process of some damage but also, importantly a process of repair that has enabled the work to continue.

Moments of Surprising Intimacy Within an Estranged Setting

While accepting the loss and limitations of working online, I have found that in this setting there have been surprising times of intimacy. When the internet connectivity fails or freezes, it can be very difficult, sometimes alarming, frustrating, or confusing for both patient and therapist. We are then left sometimes for a minute or more, looking at the patient or couple frozen in time, and they are left looking at us. I have been struck by what these images convey and sometimes feeling I am seeing something, that might have passed me by or been hidden in rapid movements had they been in person.

At other times, states of mind can be expressed or acted out through the technology, problems in connecting, sudden disconnections, muting, the placing of the device and what is captured on or left out of the screen. Some of it might be a technical problem, but sometimes it is more than that. We can get so caught up in managing the technology and helping our patients to manage it, we can miss the ways in which it is being used to communicate particular states of mind.

For example, the partners in one couple, for various reasons, were joining the session from different computers in different locations. At one particular moment in the session, one of them suddenly disconnected. My fantasy (and the partner's) was that she had metaphorically 'walked out of the room.' Whether or not she had unconsciously hit a button that cut her off, it was a dramatic moment in the session for both of them (and for me). I am not sure I would have known how unbearable what was being discussed was for her unless this had happened.

And of course, in some ways, we have more access to our patients as many give us access to their home environment. One young patient, whose relationships had irretrievably broken down, gave me an unintended tour of their apartment while she was trying to place her computer somewhere with a better connection. But was it a distraction or was it helpful information? Was it intentional on her behalf or not? I understood it in many ways, on one level I experienced it as a chaotic tour of her internal world and her feeling of not being able to settle internally following the loss of her relationship. In another more concrete way, I thought she was showing me the loved apartment and all the memories to which she was saying farewell. I also felt she was expressing her disturbance in no longer having the contained and reliable space of my room, on which she had come to depend. Thus, I have come to think that many of these strange online encounters, including technical glitches, are part of the material that can be very useful to engage with.

While patients might find it harder to bring their difficult feelings on Zoom, I have noticed that for some, the distanced feeling of Zoom has created some more intimacy with me. One couple had found it very difficult talking about sex in the room with me. They had stopped having sex some time ago, following the revelation of his affair with a work colleague. There is a lot of shame in sex for both of them, which had contributed to their sexual relationship being unsatisfactory. Since we have been working online, I have been struck by how much they have been able to talk about it and being able to do so has increased their trust and intimacy with me. We have understood that working online makes them feel more separate from me, but in a way that then allows them to increase the intimacy with me. This in essence, is the problem they have been struggling with in their sexual relationship, how it is only when they can feel separate enough that intimacy becomes possible.

Conclusion

In working online in this way, we and our patients have had to manage many difficult things, the most significant feels to me to be the changes in the external setting and the impact of not being able to meet in person. For some patients and analysts, we must acknowledge that the changes to the external setting, to use Bridge's phrase, have been "stretched too far." But when it is possible for the analyst's internal setting to be maintained or repaired and re-found, these changes in the external setting become part of the material which the analyst takes in, makes sense of, and interprets in the process of containing the patient or couple. I wouldn't advocate or choose to work on Zoom, but I have found that some of the material that is evoked in the patient or couple by this new compromised frame has been an interesting and important part of the therapeutic process, which needs to be incorporated in the process of understanding the patient or couple.

As I described earlier, during the pandemic and lockdown, many couples struggled with issues of managing the tension between closeness and what can feel claustrophobic, and then, in their dynamic, it leads to a hostile move away from relating or to estrangement. For those who have been confined to working at home together, their separate lives and interests are not available to them as they were before to help create needed physical and psychic space in their relationship.

For the analyst and the couple, the feeling of estrangement has to be managed, and within that, there are, I believe, moments of real and unexpected intimacy and connectivity. However, I think we have to accept that in this way of working, something important is missing. Perhaps when the patient gave me a tour of her apartment, she was also conveying the important and missing process of coming to her session. In face-to-face work, there is a journey, a negotiation of space in coming and going, the observation of familiar objects, the tactile experience of the setting, the familiar sounds and smells. These accumulate to provide a richness of human contact that has only become clear in its absence.

Many people, perhaps everyone, has become to some extent sadder over this long period and I believe that is because those moments of connectivity that would otherwise be considered merely background, are actually very important to us—both analyst and patient. As we move back to face-to-face working, perhaps a lot of the difficult feelings that have been managed by patients during this pandemic—sadness, depression, loss, and anger—present and need to be worked through. And I suspect that though it has been possible to work remotely and even to do good work some of the time, some of these feelings have waited for the re-establishment of the in-person analytic setting in which they can be safely expressed and contained.

References

Bridge, M., Moving out—Disruption and repair to the internal setting. British Journal of Psychotherapy 29: 481–493, 2013.

Britton, R., The missing link: Parental sexuality in the Oedipus complex. In: J. Steiner (Ed.), The Oedipus Complex Today: Clinical Implications (pp. 83–101). London: Karnac, 1989.

Churcher, J., Keeping the psychoanalytic setting in mind. Paper given to the Annual Conference of Lancaster Psychotherapy Clinic in collaboration with the Tavistock Clinic, at St Martin's College, Lancaster, 9 September 2005. An earlier version was given to the Fourteenth Annual General Meeting of the Hallam Institute for Psychotherapy, Sheffield, 8 May 2004. Available at: www.academia.edu/4527520/

Civitarese, G., Fire at the theatre: (Un)reality of/in the transference and interpretation. The International Journal of Psychoanalysis 85(5).

Cohen, J., *The Guardian Review*, Sunday March 2021, Issue No. 165, 2021.

Colman, W., The intolerable other: The difficulty in becoming a couple. Couple and Family Psychoanalysis 4(1): 22–41, 2014. (Previously published [2005] without the author's "Afterword" in Psychoanalytic Perspectives on Couple Work, 1: 56–71.).

Freud, S., Civilization and Its Discontents. The Standard Edition of the Complete Psychological Works of Sigmund Freud (Volume 21, pp. 57–146). London: Hogarth Press, 1930.

Morgan, M., A Couple State of Mind: Psychoanalysis of Couples and the Tavistock Relationships Model. London & New York: Routledge, 2019.

Morgan, M., First contacts: The therapist's "couple state of mind" as a factor in the containment of couples seen for initial consultations. In: F. Grier (Ed.), Brief Encounters with Couples (pp. 17–32). London: Karnac, 2001.

Parsons, M., Raiding the inarticulate: The internal analytic setting and listening beyond countertransference. International Journal of Psychoanalysis, 88(6): 1441–1456, 2007.

Puget, J., South American perspective. In: T. Keogh & E. Palacios (Eds.), Interpretation in Couple and Family Psychoanalysis: Cross Cultural Perspectives. London and New York: Routledge, 2019.

Winnicott, D.W., The Maturational Processes and the Facilitating Environment: Studies in the Theory of Emotional Development (pp. 29–36). London: Karnac, 1958.

Chapter 18

Distance, Fear and Intimacy in COVID Time

Gila Ofer

This chapter is written with much hesitancy and trepidation. My thoughts on the consequences of the plague we are all still experiencing change frequently. I do not know if and how the world will change, and I do not know how we will change as human beings and as therapists. And I have no certainty at all that the things I write now will seem to me relevant in several months. I share with you some experiences that I am going through and address some issues that have been sharpened for me while working therapeutically with groups in the days of COVID-19. These thoughts guide me nowadays and allow comfort and a kind of road map.

I recently heard from an English-speaking colleague that in the English language, the word plague is used as both a noun—a rapidly spreading contagious disease that kills many people—as well as a verb denoting a psychic state in which one is deeply torn up inside by some persistent wound, trouble or distress. We can say that currently the world is plagued by four overlapping crises—the coronavirus, a climate crisis, an economic collapse and a political crisis. Early on it became evident that people with certain underlying conditions are particularly vulnerable to the virus as well as others who are more privileged. But the virus also laid bare the world's underlying conditions—a heartless economy, a failure to invest in the public good, and polarized population of poor and rich, left and right, young and old, religious and secular, black and white, etc. I am aware of my own difficulty mentalizing the too-muchness of this moment, because we are in the midst of these threatening events, we are part of it, and with not enough distance from it. While I certainly have no new language to offer, what I can do is share with you some experiences I have with groups, filtered through the lens of my own sensibility.

So, we can say that we are in the middle of what seems to be an endless worldwide traumatic event. But how do we listen and what can we hear when fellow human beings become biohazards, silent invisible forces that threaten our lives, and we recoil at home, obsessively washing our hands, losing savings and income, fearful of the violence of microbes, politicians, and police? What impact does it have when the complexity of our senses—touch,

DOI: 10.4324/9781003269649-25

unmediated looks into each other's eyes, shared laughter—is flattened? What happens when we understand that reality is always too much to digest, when the principle of asymmetric reciprocity between therapist and patient is shaken? What if trauma is not something to be uncovered from the unconscious of the patient's memory but is potentially in our midst, happening to us right here, right now. In this chapter, I relate first to some ethical and technical dilemmas that we are facing at this time of COVID-19. I then relate to some issues that I faced in working with my small groups and, finally, I address how and why I worked with large groups (conducting and teaching).

The Setting

How is it different? How do we work from distance? The passage to Zoom, telephone, and others means that technology raises resistance in therapists and patients alike. The changes and oscillations in setting are outrageous, frustrating, and tiring. The loss is great—loss of physical closeness, nuances and sensory communication, trust and the non-verbal. However, does this loss compel us to question the meaning of the setting? We have to ask ourselves what is essential in the setting. More than ever, the essential and most important elements of the framework seem to be continuity, stability, and the effort to maintain trust and connection.

Stolper and Zigenlaub (2021) discuss four central themes regarding the change of setting in pandemic time and quarantine that inhibit physical encounters: the visible and the invisible, the transition from a group conductor to a group host, the group stage of development during the transition to the Zoom format, and proximity versus distance. But even meeting face to face was affected by the pandemic. I certainly had to look for a larger room for my groups. And it was not easy to find one. My patients did not like the new space (neither did I). Still, I had to believe that the essential element of the framework is internal—our intention for the well-being of the patients, for their expansion of their inner world, of strengthening the sense of freedom. These elements are our job definition face to face or via online.

The responsibility for the setting is ours. And the question of risk is mixed with other ethical questions. Who is the one who determines whether we meet in person, with or without masks, or via Zoom? I'm in a higher risk group of infection, but patients may also be in a high-risk group. How can my inner sense of freedom exist? These issues and more are inevitable from the central question—what sustains the possibility of sustaining good therapy?

Reciprocity and Symmetry

When the pandemic first struck, we were all in a heightened state of reactivity. Lacking reliable coordinates, we didn't know where we were, let alone where we were heading. Even the gradually emerging facts were hard to metabolize: the virus is deadly and highly contagious but easily killed with soap. Asymptomatic carriers can be super-spreaders, but it is also highly unlikely that one will be infected outdoors if proper distance is maintained. It is poignant that psychoanalytic and group-analytic sessions begin these days with patients and therapists alike wanting, no, needing to know, if the other is "alright," if he is vaccinated, if he is healthy. For a long time, my Chinese patient kept asking me in the beginning of every session if I put a mask on myself when I go out.

In many ways, a feeling of threat, uncertainty, and economic anxiety are common. However, the social structures that preserve injustice and inequality work harder in times of disaster. Not all of us suffer equally from the plague, and it is not just a matter of arbitrary fate. Being able to be in isolation is a privilege. The possibility of continuing to work from home is a privilege. The possibility of avoiding overcrowded spaces and having better health services is a privilege; older age is now a big danger and young ones are more privileged.

In a different context, we are in a situation where both therapist and patient are in the same threatening and frightening reality. Uncertainty is common to both sides. How can we help from equal conditions? Reciprocity and mutual influence always exist in therapy. We always have our difficulties, defenses, and anxieties. The asymmetry is not connected to our life events, rather it is connected to our ethical intentions and the fact that we are there in order to take care of the patients. But now, this asymmetry can be shuddered and almost shattered when quite often we are in a more dangerous situation than our patients. I will relate to this later when I talk about working in small groups.

Technique

What has been changed in the technique? Is it right to do the therapy in another way when reality changed so suddenly and radically? What do we do when the group is not unified in its readiness to move into online meetings or sit with masks in the room? How do we provide the right space for our groups? In my mind, the main thing that needs to be preserved now is connection, the bond formed out of reciprocity and asymmetry. The bond that keeps the empathic, curious look, striving for human contact and emotional touch, even when there is physical distance. But, within the plague and its implications, we learn even more that psychotherapy and group analysis cannot remain neutral and out of the overall context of the lives of the people we help.

Small Groups in the Time of COVID-19

When the pandemic started, I had three analytic groups which I conducted by myself. Two are in Israel and one was abroad. I would like to share with you some of the problems that came up since the beginning of the acknowledged pandemic.

Let me start with the one which was abroad. I used to work with this group in block training four to five times a year. After five years of working together, we decided to end our analytic meetings and go on only with supervision. I was supposed to meet them for the last time in March 2020. One week before I was supposed to travel to that country, the borders of my country and their country were closed. I could not go for the final block, and I also knew that this would go on for a long time. How was I to conclude my work with this group? My decision was to have two months of consecutive weekly online meetings. Eight meetings for ending five years of working together. Of course, it was not an easy decision, but, to me, it seemed the best among other options. For half a year we worked on ending the group. We could not simply go on after that. But it was a poor option. And the anger, the rage of ending like this had to be worked through. I promised that one day, when the borders open, I will come in person to meet them in person. Until today I cannot go.

Next, I'll discuss the two groups here in Israel. As soon as we had to move to online meetings (during the lockdown), two persons in one of the groups announced that they would not attend the meetings. They cannot and would not do it. For them, it is not a proper way of meeting. I had to decide whether to give up the meetings because two out of eight will not attend. I tried to correspond with them. One was very stubborn and did not come. The other attended after some correspondence with me. I thought that maintaining the bond with most of the members was more important than keeping the whole group unified. This issue occupied much of the first meeting online. I think that all those who attended the Zoom meetings agreed that it was most important and also very meaningful. The man who attended only after I convinced him did some very important work in those meetings. However, later, when we started to meet again face-to-face, he was extremely angry with me declaring that I put too much pressure on him. Both members paid for the two months although one of them was questioning the need to pay. Still, both saw themselves as part of the group although they did not join us on the Zoom meetings.

Still, there are questions to address: Should people who do not agree to attend Zoom meetings pay for them? Who decides whether to meet online or face-to-face? What can we do with patients who refuse to be vaccinated?

Large Groups in the Time of COVID-19

Until recently, large group theory in older publications describes the chaotic-aggressive, near-psychosis character of the large group, a certain contrast between the seemingly "benign" small group and the "destructive" large group and a predominantly dyadic relationship between the conductor and the large group. More recent publications underline the creative-constructive potential of the large group and the intersubjective interweaving of the conductor and the large group. Now, the main emphasis from this perspective is on promoting this potential and on the importance of communication and dialogue between the conductors and the participants, even in large groups. The analytic attitude and intervention technique would be changed (Ofer 2020, 2021): the traditional position of strict neutrality, anonymity and abstinence as well as the emphasis on whole-group interpretations would be substituted by encouragement of dialogue and by a more-open stance that does not hide the subjectivity of the conductor(s), but rather uses the conductor's subjectivity to promote the analytic process.

On the day that we heard of the COVID-19 lockdown, of the terrible situation in Italy and in Spain, I called a colleague of mine and asked him to join me in conducting a large group for the delegates and the members of all institutes of the European Federation for Psychoanalytic Psychotherapy (EFPP). I had a feeling that in this time when almost the whole world is in lockdown, when borders among countries are closed, there would be a great need for connecting and this could be one of the best ways to do it. Borders are closed, but there are holes in the closed borders. Technologies create these holes which are so important for our well-being. I took some time (procedural issues) and we started on the first Sunday of April 2020. Within a couple of minutes, we had 100 participants. Then I started receiving emails from people all over Europe asking to get in; we unfortunately could not let them in because at that time we were still limited to no more than 100 people. However, there was so much excitement in the meeting. At first, it was very formal and most of the people who were talking were Italian. But toward the end, it was very emotional—stories about dead friends and colleagues; lots of associations, anxieties, and even a dream about Noah's ark in the storm. Everybody was concerned mainly about people in Italy and Spain. There were also questions regarding behavior in the large group.

Our interventions were mainly "holding" interventions, inviting participants to add and relate, explanations regarding administration. One interpretation was to comment about the impotence of political leaders, comparing it to the impotence of the conductors of the large group who could not allow more than 100 people to the group space.

But we learned and from then on we could hold up to 500 participants. For the next eight sessions we had more and more participants on each meeting. On each session, we had participants from 21 countries in Europe. There was a solid core of participants on all meetings, but there were others who came for just a couple of meetings. There were people who could hardly speak English and others translated for them. In the beginning, there was fear of stronger emotions, but people slowly became freer in their expression of various emotions—loneliness, grief, anger, rage, etc. Some aggression among participants came up. Sometimes I did not react immediately, waiting for participants to balance each other. And then the central topic of the fear of riots came up. In the fourth session, one participant shared thoughts that she said she did not dare to say even in her individual therapy—thinking that the virus is evolutionally important and "cleaning the species" in a way that is good for humanity.

In the next meeting, people were even more open and shared personal mourning of parents, catastrophic dreams, fear of the future, and helplessness. Participants balanced each other so that after these shared concerns, a man brought some optimism to the group: on the seventh meeting, one participant told the group about his 90-year-old mother who told him that she does not understand where he disappears every Sunday evening and wonders if he is going to Paris! The story, content and way of telling it brought liveliness and vitality to the group. We now had Eros in the group. Participants, especially women, talked about the perfumes they put on for the meetings. We could almost smell through the web! One member from Russia told us that following this large group, another one was started in Russia for those who do not understand English. And others from other countries also told us about similar groups following us. The last meetings dealt with the ending of this group and asking for more meetings. It was very exciting when many of the participants brought with them flowers and showed them in the Zoom windows for appreciation for our work. I felt that this large group was most important for those who participated and offered a space for sharing, expressing emotions, love, and most of all, communicating and psychic touching where the virus, social distancing, and closed borders could not make those possible.

The need for large groups was also felt by me when I decided, together with a colleague, to give a course on conducting large groups to group analysts. We decided to teach it online to a group of 15 people. Within a couple of days, we had more than 30 people on the list. The participants were asked to attend large groups that were running at that time, and were given theoretical papers to read. This course was successful and was another testimony for the need for such groups on pandemic times.

Concluding Remarks

As I mentioned in the opening, we are now faced with a three poles pandemic: health, economic and political. Now, for some individuals, breakdown feels imminent. This fear of catastrophe might be a prescient intuition of what is to come or an unconscious draw toward a catastrophe. We may feel a degree of panic at the arbitrariness of fate; yet most of us also have a sense of being among people, if not national leaders, who can protect us. In my country, I saw it in the demonstrations that took place all over the country, and the change of government. Although our lives may never be quite the same, let us speak at least as much about our fundamental resilience, our creativity, and our tendency to communicate. In psychoanalysis, we praise interdependence. We need each other because omnipotence doesn't really keep us safe. The ease with which this virus is transmitted compels us to face how interdependent we really are.

Personally, I am more inclined to hope than to desire. Desire means that there is only one way to reach what is needed. Hope is not the conviction that things will turn out well, but the belief that things can make sense, regardless of how they turn out. "We've got to be as clear headed about human beings as possible," says the writer James Baldwin, "because we are still each other's only hope." We are each other's only hope because the damage humans inflict upon each other is far greater than what this virus can do. And because we can only really think when we have others to think with. This is why groups at this time are so important.

Especially during a plague, we need to keep each other alive and sustain each other's aliveness. At a time of social distancing, we need to find common purpose in response to necessity. And to remind each other that even if people die, we can't exhaust the human heart.

Reference

Ofer, G. Distance and intimacy in COVID-19 time. Lecture given at the EFPP conference Pandemic in Our Life: impact on our patients, 2021.

Ofer, G., The impact of COVID-19 on Working with Groups. Lecture given to the community of mental health professionals in Istanbul, 2020.

Stolper, E. & Zigenlaub, E., From the Circle to the Square: Group Psychotherapy in the Age of Corona Virus. *Group*, 45(1), 2021.

Thanks

To all the contributors who have made possible this book.

To Hansjorg Messner and Ulrich-Venrath Schulz, my co-editors, for our most appreciated work as a team, moving forward even when it seemed difficult.

To Anna Maria Nicolò for her beautiful and complete introduction to this book.

To Susannah Frearson, Ellie Duncan, Singhania Saloni, Jana Craddock and all the rest of the Routledge team for their professional support, patience and amazing skills.

To Michael Buchholz and Aleksandar Dimitrijevic for promoting this project by providing encouraging blurbs.

To Tija Despotovic and Bojana Mitrović for their help and dedication in the first part of this project.

And the last, but not the least, a very respectful thanks to Anne-Marie Schlösser for her hard work and perseverance, patience and creativity and for help during my transition as Editor-in-Chief.

Index

Note: Page numbers followed by "n" refer to notes; and page numbers in **bold** refer to tables; and page numbers in *italics* refer to figures.